ARTHRITIS, RHEUMATISM AND YOUR ACHING BACK

ARTHRITIS, RHEUMATISM AND YOUR ACHING BACK

by J. I. Rodale

and the Staff of *Prevention*

RODALE BOOKS, INC.

Emmaus, Penna. 18049

Standard Book Number 87596-045-6
Library of Congress Catalog Card Number 79-104179

PRINTED IN THE UNITED STATES
G-43
First Printing—June, 1970

Table of Contents

CHAPTER I

Is A Cure Possible?

JUST ABOUT any doctor will tell you that arthritis and rheumatism are incurable. In the entire multi-billion dollar armament of pills and capsules stored in drug companies and corner pharmacy shelves across the country, there is not one drug—not one!—that can cure the major rheumatic diseases.

Yet, strange as it may seem, a great number of people have testified to being "cured" of arthritis and rheumatism through a wide variety of methods unassociated with drugs. Certainly what has worked for one of them will not necessarily work for all others. Nonetheless, here are some of their own personal experiences:

"I had arthritis for 11 years. The crippling kind, rheumatoid arthritis. I spent a lot of money on it, including $500 at one doctor's office, and guess what completely cured me? Alfalfa tea, 4 or 5 glasses a day, every day. I had it so bad it put me on crutches at times. Now this is made with the seed, not the leaves."

—A. Grant, Illinois

"I have the arthritis so bad in my shoulders and arms, back and hips, but in your magazine I learned about vitamins. I sent away for the Preventive Project of five bottles: bone meal, rose hips, E complex, desiccated liver and yeast concentrate and also dolomite A & D tablets. The pain was so bad I could not lay down in bed it hurt my shoulders so, and I had to take aspirin. But now I don't have to, and I can lay down all night, and my arms, shoulders and back are so much better. If it had not been for your magazine I would never have known about them. My doctor did tell me to take vitamin B_{12}. I think they did help some, but I have gotten much better since I have taken the others."

—Mrs. Mable Y., New York

"I would like to tell your readers how I solved my arthritis problem. I had this disease in the spine, elbow and fingers. Since taking a combination tablet of calcium, magnesium, vitamin A and D, plus vitamin C, I no longer have pain. I was told by a nutritionist that this combination helps to build up the cartilage between the bones, and it is also good for broken bones—they heal faster. It takes about two weeks for your system to saturate itself with this combination. Then, wham! The pain is gone."

—Mrs. Mabel G., Alaska

"My case is a proof of what the May issue of your magazine says about curing arthritis. In the 20's I had a serious case of rheumatoid arthritis. The acute state wore off, leaving me crippled and weak. My joints were not ankylosed, however, until my tonsils were removed. After that, exercises which were temporarily helpful, were no longer effective. My back was badly bent, I could not take a deep breath, knees and hips were bent, and shoulders so fixed that I could not put my hands on my hips. I had a rigid neck.

"In 1933, I was lucky enough to be recommended to a doctor who, little by little, broke up the ankylosis and also gave me a proper diet. . . .

"Well, I became more and more active, finally took some summer courses and went back to teaching. At 65 I completed eight more years as a full time teacher. I am now in good health."

—Helen J., Massachusetts

"Last winter arthritis came upon me until it was painful to get up, get in and out of the car, and bending down was too much to attempt.

"I read in *Prevention* that arthritis could be

helped from a reader who had suffered, with no help from drugs, so the same plan was followed by me. I took four bone meal tablets with each meal and in one week every pain was gone and I could exercise with no trouble.

"No doubt the vitamins and food supplements that I have taken during the past years helped to condition my system, but how wonderful it is to enjoy being free of all pain."

—Arthur W., Massachusetts

"They say one is never really cured but I don't agree at all. I had a very bad case of arthritis in 1951. My elbows and knees were swollen very bad and my fingers were so swollen that my wedding ring had to be cut off. I haven't had a trace of it since. Now if this isn't a sign that I am cured I don't know what more proof I would need.

"I had it so bad I was in the hospital for about two weeks I couldn't even use my fingers much. I went back to my doctor for regular check-ups. I haven't been back for about two years.

"My doctor told me that I would always have it.

"I do take bone meal, yeast tablets, wheat germ, and vitamins. I would just like to have people know that there is a cure. I am positive. And if I could help other people this would make me happy. I am a widow, 58 years old and work about seven months a year.

"Thank you so much."

—Mrs. Betty J., Iowa

These people are not talking about any supernatural miracles. But they are talking about significant improvements and possibly cures. They are telling us that, although orthodox medicine tells them drugs can offer little lasting hope, they have found that hope indeed exists.

That is what this book is about.

CHAPTER II

You Are Not Alone

IF YOU are suffering from rheumatic disease, you are certainly not alone. Virtually all animal life has travailed at one time or another in the agonies of arthritis and the other rheumatoid diseases. Perhaps 200 million years ago, when giant animals stalked the earth, rheumatoid diseases plagued their muscles and bones. Recently discovered skeletons of the mighty dinosaurs show that even they were victims of the muscle and skeletal diseases. Bones of the forerunner of the horse, the eohippus, show that it, too, suffered rheumatic diseases.

Those diseases, primarily falling into the general classifications rheumatism and arthritis, found a whole new host of victims with the advent of man. The Java ape man certainly suffered, according to scientists who have studied skeletal remains.

The Neanderthal man probably did, too. In the days of the Pharaohs, arthritis was probably as common as it is today. Mummified Egyptians bear testimony to that fact.

And through each age, rheumatic disease has plagued new victims. It crippled the Romans, the Norman invaders, the great kings of Europe, scientists, philosophers, explorers, the Puritans, the American Indians.

It has advanced side by side with medical science, so that Robert Bingham, M.D., a California orthopedic surgeon, reported at an Annual Seminar of the American Nutrition Society in 1967 that today the rheumatoid diseases have struck one out of every 20 persons in the United States and Canada. "Rheumatism and arthritis are more common than the total number of cases of tuberculosis, diabetes, cancer and heart disease combined," he said. "Arthritis surpasses injury from accidents. From the standpoint of days lost from work and in the older age groups it is the chief cause of forced retirement."

According to a Public Affairs Committee report, the total number of American victims of rheumatoid diseases is as great as the total population of the state of Texas. Of the 12 million estimated to be ill, 250,000 are completely disabled. Ninety-seven per cent of all those living beyond the age of 35 undergo changes in the bones and joints which are indicative of arthritis. About one in ten of these people actually suffer symptoms.

Exact statistics are difficult to come by. According to the American Rheumatism Association, "Knowledge of the prevalence of rheumatic disease is at present inexact and confused because of the practical limitations of the completed surveys and the lack of generally accepted criteria defining the diseases included." But according to the United States National Health Survey completed in June, 1959, an estimated 10,845,000 persons were reported to have arthritis or rheumatism, a rate of approximately 6.4 per cent. This ranged from 0.2 per cent of persons under 25 years of age to 28.6 per cent of persons 75 years and older. Of note was the fact that 42 per cent were not under medical care at the time of the interview, while a further 19 per cent had never been medically attended.

But the fact that the rheumatic diseases are on the increase was illustrated in an updated report on their prevalence in May, 1968. The Arthritis Foundation said then, "New survey figures which put the number of people in the U.S. suffering some form of arthritis at 16.8 million are revealed in the annual report of the Arthritis Foundation. This is an increase of more than three and a half million over previous estimates of the country's arthritis population. Since the total population of the country is now more than 200 million, it means that one in 11 people have arthritis. The old figure was one in 16."

The rheumatic diseases cause an incredible

amount of absenteeism. More than 115 million work-days are lost annually because of these diseases—the equivalent of 470,000 persons out of work for the entire year. The cost to industry is equally incredible—more than one billion five hundred million dollars annually. Even Uncle Sam suffers. In taxes he loses 200 million dollars each year, and he pays out almost that much annually in subsistence allowances to arthritics who are not able to support themselves.

Around the world, private nonprofit organizations are also contributing millions of dollars toward research in the rheumatic diseases. There are 40 countries with professional rheumatism societies. The largest of these, with 1,600 members is the American Rheumatism Association, founded in 1934. Each year it brings the world's leading experts together to discuss their new findings and plan new approaches.

Private organizations have also been organized to combat the rheumatic diseases. In the United States, the Arthritis and Rheumatism Foundation was founded in 1948, and similar organizations exist in 13 countries. Their members have contributed countless hours and dollars to eliminate the rheumatic diseases.

But there is no question who pays the most to fight arthritis. The victims themselves do. Financially, medical expenses for arthritis and rheumatism total one billion dollars a year, according to the Arthritis Foundation's 20th annual report in

1967. The figure is enormous, but it does not suggest the poverty to which some poor arthritis victims have been subjected in order to find relief from their suffering. For the rheumatoid diseases—with the exception of rheumatic fever—rarely kill. Instead, they torture. To escape the pain, many a person of modest means has spent his life savings in vain.

For that reason, the rheumatoid diseases are as tragic as—and perhaps more tragic than—many of those which take the victim's life outright.

The average person would undoubtedly have a difficult time defining the terms "rheumatic disease," "rheumatism" and "arthritis." The confusion over these terms is nothing to be ashamed of—most doctors are hard-put to define them, and even an expert in these diseases recently found himself constantly contradicting his own statements in trying to supply an adequate definition. "Well, we in the profession know what we're talking about even if we can't explain it to outsiders," he finally shrugged.

This book is about the "rheumatic diseases," a general term which means, simply, symptoms of pain in the musculo-skeletal system. As we have said, the rheumatic diseases are divided into two major categories: rheumatism and arthritis.

Rheumatism is no more scientific a term, however, than stomach trouble. It refers only to aches and pains which begin at certain joints in the body, but also extend into the muscular tissue, tendons, nerves and connective tissues. Just as the grand and almost meaningless topic "stomach trouble" could include anything from ulcers to acid indigestion, so "rheumatism" can include a world of diverse problems. For that reason, doctors seldom use the term in professional discussions.

Among the more common forms of rheumatism are bursitis, fibrositis, neuritis, lumbago, sciatica, myositis, fascitis, tenosynovitis and tendinitis. Each of them are distinct diseases, and we will discuss them in later chapters.

Arthritis is a far more meaningful word than rheumatism. Medically, the body's joints are called "articulations." In medical lingo, the suffix "-itis" means inflammation. Obviously, therefore, "arthritis" is inflammation of a joint. It is interesting to realize that arthritis, at least according to the professionals, is not a disease. It is a sign of a disease —a symptom which suggests that a disease is present.

That is one of the many reasons for the confusion in defining the rheumatoid diseases. Arthritis, considered one of the major rheumatoid diseases, is not truly a disease after all!

The following classification breakdown of Arthritis and Rheumatism drawn up by the American Rheumatism Association is the most clear-cut and systematic available. But the Association is quick to point out that it is only tentative. A discovery concerning causation of any of the disorders could easily disrupt the classification table.

PRIMER ON RHEUMATIC DISEASES

ARA Nomenclature and Classification of Arthritis and Rheumatism (Tentative)

I. Polyarthritis of unknown etiology
  A. Rheumatoid arthritis
  B. Juvenile rheumatoid arthritis (Still's disease)
  C. Ankylosing spondylitis
  D. Psoriatic arthritis
  E. Reiter's syndrome
  F. Others

II. "Connective tissue" disorders
  A. Systemic lupus erythematosus
  B. Polyarteritis nodosa
  C. Scleroderma (progressive systemic sclerosis)
  D. Polymyositis and dermatomyositis
  E. Others

III. Rheumatic fever

IV. Degenerative joint disease (osteoarthritis, osteoarthrosis)
  A. Primary
  B. Secondary

V. Nonarticular rheumatism
  A. Fibrositis
  B. Intervertebral disc and low back syndromes
  C. Myositis and myalgia
  D. Tendinitis and peritendinitis (bursitis)
  E. Tenosynovitis
  F. Fasciitis
  G. Carpal tunnel syndrome
  H. Others
  (See also shoulder-hand syndrome, VIII. E.)

VI. Diseases with which arthritis is frequently associated
  A. Sarcoidosis
  B. Relapsing polychondritis
  C. Henoch-Schönlein syndrome
  D. Ulcerative colitis
  E. Regional ileitis
  F. Whipple's disease
  G. Sjögren's syndrome
  H. Familial Mediterranean fever
  I. Others
  (See also psoriatic arthritis, I.D.)

VII. Associated with known infectious agents
  A. Bacterial
    1. Brucella
    2. Gonococcus
    3. Mycobacterium tuberculosis
    4. Pneumococcus
    5. Salmonella
    6. Staphylococcus
    7. Streptobacillus moniliformis (Haverhill fever)
    8. Treponema pallidum (syphilis)
    9. Treponema pertenue (yaws)
    10. Others
  B. Rickettsial
  C. Viral
  D. Fungal
  E. Parasitic
  (See also rheumatic fever, III.)

VIII. Traumatic and/or neurogenic disorders
  A. Traumatic arthritis (viz, the result of direct trauma)
  B. Lues (tertiary syphilis)
  C. Diabetes
  D. Syringomyelia
  E. Shoulder-hand syndrome
  F. Mechanical derangement of joints
  G. Others
  (See also degenerative joint disease, IV.; carpal tunnel syndrome, V.G.)

IX. Associated with known biochemical or endocrine abnormalities
  A. Gout
  B. Ochronosis
  C. Hemophilia
  D. Hemoglobinopathies (eg, sickle cell disease)
  E. Agammaglobulinemia
  F. Gaucher's disease
  G. Hyperparathyroidism
  H. Acromegaly
  I. Hypothyroidism
  J. Scurvy (hypovitaminosis C)
  K. Xanthoma tuberosum
  L. Others
  (See also multiple myeloma, X.G.; Hurler's syndrome, XII.C.)

X. Tumor and tumor-like conditions
  A. Synovioma
  B. Pigmented villonodular synovitis
  C. Giant cell tumor of tendon sheath
  D. Primary juxta-articular bone tumors
  E. Metastatic
  F. Leukemia
  G. Multiple myeloma

PRIMER ON RHEUMATIC DISEASES

ARA Nomenclature and Classification of Arthritis and Rheumatism (Tentative)

- H. Benign tumors of articular tissue
- I. Others

(See also hypertrophic osteoarthropathy, XIII.G.)

XI. Allergy and drug reactions
- A. Arthritis due to specific allergens (eg, serum sickness)
- B. Arthritis due to drugs (eg, hydralazine syndrome)
- C. Others

XII. Inherited and congenital disorders
- A. Marfan's syndrome
- B. Ehlers-Danlos syndrome
- C. Hurler's syndrome
- D. Congenital hip dysplasia
- E. Morquio's disease
- F. Others

XIII. Miscellaneous disorders
- A. Amyloidosis
- B. Aseptic necrosis of bone
- C. Behcet's syndrome
- D. Chondrocalcinosis (pseudogout)
- E. Erythema multiforme (Stevens-Johnson syndrome)
- F. Erythema nodosum
- G. Hypertrophic osteoarthropathy
- H. Juvenile osteochondritis
- I. Osteochondritis dissecans
- J. Reticulohistiocytosis of joints (lipoid dermato-arthritis)
- K. Tietze's disease
- L. Others

That is the major problem in defining the rheumatic diseases—so little is known about them. (The irony is that the diseases have been around and caused suffering for so long, and so much time and money has been spent trying to learn more about them.)

We have said that arthritis is a symptom of disease, not the disease itself. We have known for a long time, for example, that venereal disease often produces arthritis as a side effect. Infection of the joints is a frequent development of gonorrhea cases between 5 and 30 days after infection. The pain customarily comes on suddenly, affecting many body joints, and is accompanied by fever. Within a few days, pain localizes in the knee, elbow, wrist or ankle. The standard treatment for gonorrhea—penicillin—is usually effective in clearing up gonococcal arthritis.

Viruses other than those associated with venereal diseases are known to cause arthritis. Those which cause mumps, influenza and epidemic hepatitis are known to produce short-term arthritis attacks. The virus most frequently guilty, however, is the rubella (measles) virus. Young adults are often affected, especially females, and the arthritis persists for two to 14 days.

Tuberculosis-caused arthritis, while declining in the United States, is still the most common form of chronic infectious arthritis. It develops in approximately four per cent of patients who have other forms of tuberculosis. Indeed, there are instances in which arthritis may be a blessing in disguise. Occasionally tuberculosis symptoms are so obscure that it could go unnoticed until it reached serious proportions. Only the obvious pain of arthritis leads in those cases to detailed investigation for tuberculosis.

These are examples of arthritis caused by infections. A blow or injury—trauma, as a doctor would say—can also lead to arthritis. Ask anyone who has ever dropped a heavy weight on his hand, for example. Chances are good he is now suffering from arthritis in that hand.

Gout is also considered a form of arthritis. It is one of the few forms that is today completely curable. Rheumatic fever is also related to arthritis insofar as arthritis can be caused by rheumatic fever.

The two most common and serious forms of arthritis are osteoarthritis and rheumatoid arthritis. The symptoms are similar in each: pain, heat, redness, swelling, and crippling. The commonest as well as the most ravaging is rheumatoid arthritis. It starts with a general feeling of fatigue, soreness, stiffness and aching before localized symptoms begin to appear. The joints of the hands and feet are most likely to be affected, and gradually they lose their ability to move freely. Lumps or nodules may appear under the skin. The eyes may become inflamed. Anemia or pleurisy or both may develop.

Osteoarthritis is usually a great deal less painful. Whereas rheumatoid arthritis is not uncommon in people 20 to 45 years of age, osteoarthritis is almost always associated with advancing age. Most frequently it affects the weight-bearing joints such as the knees, hips and spine. There is often no inflammation.

In following chapters we will discuss these two diseases, their causes and their treatment, the facts and the myths surrounding them. We will discuss the latest scientific attempts to treat them and cure them. But all the time we will keep in mind that modern proverb: "Science is not a sacred cow, science is a horse—don't worship it, feed it."

Many physicians, in their admirable zeal to bring relief to suffering patients, have embraced with open arms every new drug that the science labs of drug companies have turned out. Some drugs are effective in bringing relief and under certain circumstances may be wisely recommended. But that is certainly not true for every arthritis drug on the market.

Two points must be kept in mind when taking drugs for arthritis. One is that drugs never cure—they simply reduce the body's ability to recognize pain and discomfort. The same processes which ordinarily cause the suffering may still be going on, but the person with the disease doesn't recognize it.

Secondly, all drugs are toxic to a greater or lesser degree. When a drug is taken in excess, or when it is sold to the public before it is sufficiently tested, tragedy can result.

An arthritis drug called phenylbutazone was the villain in a horrifying story in the *Journal of the American Medical Association* for September 11, 1954. The author, Ephraim P. Engleman, M.D., and his associates, related the stories of six women who had been taking this drug for bursitis or arthritic pains. All the women developed hepatitis (liver disease). Two of them died, the others recovered in from 3 to 15 weeks. It is well known that hepatitis can result from blood transfusions or other injections in which the needle may not have been properly sterilized. But none of these patients had had injections. The authors conclude that it was the phenylbutazone which brought on the hepatitis and they add "hepatitis is another possible hazard in the therapeutic use of this drug." They do not state what the other hazards are, but we assume from this that there may be many others as well.

Among the latest in a long series of drugs hailed as wonder-workers is chloroquinone which started out as an antimalaria drug. A report given in *Chemical Week* for September 7, 1957, describes the work of a Canadian physician who used the drug on 125 arthritic patients over a four-year period and got, he said, good results in 71 per cent of the cases. Dr. Bagnall, the physician, considered chloroquinone an agent to control arthritis —a "major step forward"—a drug to be used perhaps in conjunction with the so-called steroid drugs like cortisone. But, 12 years later, the medical profession freely concedes that aspirin is as good as any other drug for control of arthritis—and that's not too good.

What of cortisone, the miracle drug that preceded chloroquinone? Cortisone is a substance derived from the adrenal glands, which have a lot to do with maintaining resistance to disease. Human beings and animals as well have these glands. Adrenocorticotrophin hormone or ACTH (now being used as a drug, too) is a substance made from the pituitary or master gland of the body. When ACTH is injected, it stimulates the adrenal glands to produce cortisone. When cortisone was first tried out on arthritis patients, results were astonishing. Pain disappeared, a sense of well being and a good appetite returned. However, it was soon admitted that improvement stopped as soon as treatment stopped, so cortisone was no cure. In addition it was found that, in many cases, extremely serious after-effects ensued. One of the commonest is osteoporosis, general demineralization of the bones, leaving them easy to break and hard to mend.

Patients might become disturbed mentally. They might develop abnormally round faces and abnormal growths of hair. ACTH might bring about diabetes or high blood pressure. Then, too, any slight infection becomes a menace to the patient taking these drugs, for he is not aware of the infection. If it should be tuberculosis or something equally serious, it can develop into a fatal disease rapidly, which the patient, delighted that he feels so well, overexerts himself and courts disaster.

Another side effect was revealed by a doctor whose letter appeared in *The Digest of Treatment* (October, 1951). He attributed the suicide of one of his patients to cortisone treatments. In *Modern Medicine* (May, 1954) it was pointed out that in general, within a few hours after cortisone or ACTH therapy begins, the patient experiences a feeling of irritability, restlessness, tension or emotional instability. About half pass out of this stage back to normalcy; in the rest abnormal mental changes appear by the fourth day. These manifest themselves in thinking and behavioral disturbances.

The euphoric feeling some patients get from

these drugs was found to create another problem. They could convince themselves that normally painful or alarming symptoms of disease do not exist. The *Journal of the American Geriatrics Society* (November, 1955) tells of two cases in which the symptoms of active pneumonia were completely suppressed due to treatment with cortisone. The patients continued normal routines, unaware all the while of suffering with severe pneumonia. If an examining physician had not discovered the situation by chance, the patients would probably have died. The author concluded, "It cannot be stressed too often that these drugs should be used under close supervision, for, in their present form there are far too many side effects of fatal consequence."

The ulcers and infections that crop up during cortisone and ACTH therapy are mentioned again and again in the medical journals. The damage to bones that results in easy breakage is cited in the *Scottish Medical Journal* (1958, 3:450). An asthma patient being treated with corticosteroids reported a spontaneous fracture of the femur. In the *Journal of the American Medical Association* (October 2, 1954) it is reported that four patients receiving cortisone developed multiple fractures of the spine.

Evidence of the dangers involved in the use of steroid drugs is still piling up. The *Lancet* (June 1, 1957) bluntly affirmed the fact that steroids could be a direct cause of death in themselves. Of 18 deaths associated with such therapy, the drugs were considered directly responsible in 11 cases, and probably hastened death in three or four more.

No one knows exactly how these side effects come about. But we do know that glands are powerful influences, governing all the activities of the body. Taking a hormone, any hormone, is bound to disturb the delicate balance among the glands and bring abnormalities. Cortisone and ACTH, as well as any other drugs affecting glands, should never be taken except under strictest supervision so that side effects can be detected early.

An earlier treatment of arthritis was "gold therapy." This consists of injections of a preparation of gold salts. Says Dr. Walter C. Alvarez of the Mayo Foundation in his book *How to Live With Your Arthritis* (Wilcox and Follett Company), "The drug works best in the early stages of the disease before the joints are badly damaged. The big difficulty is that the medicine can do much harm to some persons and it can even cause death. Hence it should be given only by a physician who has had enough experience with it so that he can quickly recognize the danger signals and stop."

The old story. A drug so dangerous that, in careless hands, it may be far worse than the disease it is being given to cure.

Aspirin is the drug which has been used longest to relieve the pain of arthritis. Most of us think of aspirin as just about the least harmful of all drugs.

But medical literature is full of warnings about aspirin and dire tales of what happened to people who took too much or took it too long.

Of course when we talk about aspirin we mean as well practically all the pain-killing drugs, for it forms the base of many of them. Many people are allergic to aspirin and will suffer reactions to even the smallest dosage. Aspirin is an irritant to the stomach lining, so severe an irritant that it is not advised for ulcer patients—or indeed anyone with any kind of stomach disorder. Taking aspirin for rheumatic pains over a long period of time may cause any or all of the following: nausea, heartburn, stomach pain, deafness, dizziness, ringing in the ears. Doctors generally wait for their arthritic patients who are taking aspirin to tell them that their ears are ringing before they decide to cut the dosage. That is a sign that you've had enough, or far too much, depending on how you look at it.

Aspirin may cause intestinal bleeding or hemorrhages in other parts of the body, for it destroys vitamin K and the clumping ability of the platelets, both of which aid in coagulation of the blood. It may produce bleeding or stone formation in the urine. It may bring serious trouble to patients susceptible to coronary thrombosis—it may cause death.

That, too, is a sign that you've had enough.

We mention all these symptoms to warn against the casual and prolonged taking of aspirin. The effects of the newer drugs like cortisone are usually closely watched by physicians. But we can buy aspirin at the drugstore and take as much as we want without any advice from a physician. And we do buy 10 billion aspirin tablets a year in this country, donating a total of close to $200,000,000 to the drug companies for this one item alone.

Another treatment for the rheumatic diseases is sex hormones. Sex hormones carry a threat that is certainly not fully recognized by those patients who use them freely. No one knowing the risk would chance their side effects unless there were no other choice. Some years ago Dr. Erwin E. Nelson, then medical director of the Food and Drug Administration, pointed out that sterility and even cancer of the prostate, due to stimulation of dormant cancer cells present in the prostate glands of many men, are potential dangers from the misuse of the hormone testosterone.

Dr. Nelson warned women of the danger in the use of the female hormone estrogen. Prolonged use may bring about sterility, especially in women whose natural hormone secretion is normal. The use of such drugs in pill, liquid or cosmetic lotion or cream form, is extremely hazardous.

Any hormonal treatment in pregnancy is considered to be particularly perilous: The journals warn that serious alterations in the development of the expected child can occur as the result of the mother's dosage of hormones. In the *Journal of the American Medical Association* (August 8, 1959) there was a report from a German medical magazine describing three such cases. The malformations involved the brain and the spinal cord, the lungs, the liver, spleen, intestinal muscles and bones. Careful calculations determined that the abnormal fetal development began at the same time as the estrogen treatment. Experiments with pregnant rats showing severe fetal damage after the administration of estrogens support this view.

But the popular press has continually misled the public into believing its only hope rests with drugs.

In *Look* magazine for May, 1962, we read some remarkable claims for the work of Dr. Robert Liefmann in treating arthritis. The doctor stated that he could "practically wipe out the symptoms of arthritis in one year," by using his liquid formula (a mixture including cortisone and sex hormones as its main ingredients).

No sooner had his story appeared than the Arthritis and Rheumatism Foundation descended on Dr. Liefmann, charging that his claims were unrealistic, and were in effect promising a miracle cure.

Patients who have arthritis and consult the average doctor may not be promised a miraculous cure, but they are led with false assurance into a course of treatment which, in most cases, will last a lifetime. The treatment is likely to end with an arthritic condition which makes the arthritis they began with seem mild by comparison. The side effects of the drugs that are likely to be used in the course of treatment are rarely mentioned, and still more rarely, seriously considered.

In more fortunate cases, the reactions are minor

—sometimes even humorous. For example, the arthritis drug chloroquine can make a blond out of you. An interesting side effect has been noticed by some users of this drug for rheumatoid arthritis—it bleaches the hair. One writer in the *British Medical Journal* for August 4, 1956, had come across two such cases within six months of starting the drug. Both ladies became universally blond, even to the eyebrows. Luckily the change in pigmentation did not disturb either of the women emotionally, but what the drug did to the rest of their systems, if it could bleach hair, is something we may never know.

By no means are we saying that all drugs are useless against arthritis and the other rheumatic diseases. There is ample evidence that some drugs combat the pain, and a few even have minimal side effects. But the great enthusiasm with which some medical practitioners abandon themselves to drug therapy for the rheumatic diseases indicates that often these drugs prove to be the most current plateau in the evolutionary development of quackery and arthritis therapy.

That development is not surprising. For, as old as arthritis is, quack cures are just as old. According to New York State Department of Health Commissioner Hollis S. Ingraham, "Quackery is as old as mankind. I suppose the first quack was the serpent in the Garden of Eden. 'Eat of the fruit of the Tree of Knowledge,' he said, 'and you will be smart.'

(1) They note that they have only a limited amount of time to give patients, and feel they can spend their time better treating ones they can help than the others. (2) They feel that they have not been adequately trained to treat rheumatic diseases—and they are right. (3) They admit that they get more satisfaction out of treating patients who can eventually improve than they do in treating a long-term disease such as arthritis. In the words of science writer Blair Justice, "Arthritis in short, is not an 'in' disease. It is not dramatic or glamorous. There are no 'heroes' among doctors who treat arthritis as there are among surgeons who may 'cure' cancer."

But even if the average physician would be concerned for the many arthritis victims who will inevitably make their way to his office, and even if he was willing to dedicate the time needed to treat each one of them, the stark truth remains that medical science today has very little to offer. In spite of the drugs, in spite of the advice, there is not a great deal of lasting value that even the best trained and most dedicated physician can do along orthodox medical lines to help his arthritic patients. In spite of the untold millions of dollars already spent on research, medical science simply does not have the answers.

Yet, reports appear periodically in the medical literature dealing with individual research projects on the causes, treatment and cure of arthritis. The findings are often of an unorthodox nature—

which means, simply, that they do not agree with majority opinion. The difference between these findings and quackery is the difference between night and day. The quack, we have said, is "an ignorant or fraudulent pretender to medical skill." These researchers are among the best trained men in the world. They have no ax to grind, nothing to gain by their findings except the assurance that they have helped mankind. Frequently their colleagues totally ignore their findings, with the possible result that a solution to the problem of rheumatic diseases may have gone totally unnoticed. But, whereas medical science recognizes its inability to cope adequately with the rheumatic diseases, some of these unorthodox investigators feel that they have met with varying degrees of success.

In the following chapters we will discuss findings of some of the investigators whose research offers hope to the arthritic.

CHAPTER III

Osteoarthritis

IN ITS 1967 annual report, the Arthritis Foundation poignantly described the tragedy of arthritis and its treatment by modern medicine:

"A human life in crisis, saved by some heroic action or daring procedure . . . this is drama, and the world takes notice.

"A discovery that eliminates a 'killer' disease and prolongs man's life span is drama . . . and the world takes notice.

"The legislator voting a public health appropriation, the contributor deciding priorities for his health charity dollar, the administrator devising a medical school curriculum or the news editor choosing a medical story . . . each is influenced by the drama of life versus death.

"Even the physician ministering to the sick is not immune to the tug of drama when a shot or a pill produces an overnight recovery in his patient.

"But with arthritis there is little drama. And the world takes little notice.

"Arthritis is slow misery. Everything about it is gradual . . . the way it comes on . . . the way it gets worse. Even when treatment works, it can take weeks for improvement to be noticeable. The word doctors use for it is 'long-term.'

"In numbers of sufferers and in economic losses, arthritis outranks the killer diseases and most other health problems.

"But in competition for public concern and public action, it still ranks in the never-never land of the also-ran.

"There is the paradox.

"For despite the 'explosive' growth of rheumatology, despite the new interest and increasing numbers of people involved, despite the surging activity and accomplishment in every facet of the arthritis fight, it is still possible to say with accuracy today most of the negative things that were voiced in 1948.

"*The same words still apply* . . . apathy . . . indifference . . . neglect . . . ignorance . . . pessimism . . . hopelessness.

"*It is still true that the national dollar investment against arthritis is pitifully small.*

"As the population has increased, the number of arthritis sufferers in the country has more than doubled in twenty years. The latest figures . . . attest vividly to an incongruous disparity . . . a disease with a staggering impact on society being assigned by that society an absurdly low priority for attention.

"It is still true that many medical schools offer the undergraduate student little or no training in the rheumatic diseases.

"Only slightly more than half the medical schools in the United States have given the rheumatic diseases a prominent place in their curricula, many having done so only in recent years.

"The longer a physician has been out of medical school, the less likely he is to have been exposed to arthritis problems in school and to have been trained in dealing with them.

"It is still true that the majority of practicing physicians do not know how to treat arthritis to prevent disability.

"No doctor should ever say, 'You have arthritis and there is not much that can be done for you; take aspirin and don't bother to come back.' But many doctors do. . . ."

Yes, many doctors do.

Ten years ago Karl Lutz, a Pittsburgh patent attorney, began to develop arthritis. It is not unusual. Karl was 62 years old. Almost everyone that age suffers in one degree or another from arthritis.

The difference between Karl and the others was that he was not willing to resign himself to life as an invalid. Even in the early stages of the disease he found that he couldn't lift his arm above his shoulder. Sleeping was difficult, and he frequently had to cope with the kind of pain only arthritics know about. Karl reasoned that if he could correct the problem while it was still a minor one, he might be able to free himself from the disease.

His doctor offered no hope. "Yes, Karl, you have arthritis," he said. "But there's nothing we can do to cure it. My advice to you is to go on just as you are. When your condition grows worse, we can begin treating it to reduce some of the pain."

Karl Lutz didn't need a doctor to tell him to sit back and do nothing. He began searching on his own for an answer, acquiring books and medical journals which dealt with the subject. None of those he came across offered any help.

Three months after Karl visited his doctor, he attended a convention for patent lawyers in Boston. There he met an old friend, a chemical patent lawyer. As they chatted, the friend took some capsules from his pocket and swallowed them.

"What are they?" Karl asked.

"These?" the friend asked, taking a tiny container from his pocket. "These are the answer to my arthritis problem." Then he told Karl that for years he had been suffering from arthritis. He found, as Karl had, that modern medicine could offer nothing but relief from pain, and even that relief was only partial, temporary and often obtained at the cost of the body's general well-being.

Karl's friend had found that his particular type of arthritis was a disease caused by deficiency of certain nutrients, and he had begun replacing those nutrients by taking certain vitamin and mineral supplements regularly.

The idea made sense to Karl. Before turning to law, he had graduated with a degree in biochemistry, and had learned that the body needs 40 to 45 nutrients in proper balance daily if it is to be healthy. "It has been said so often it is almost trite," Karl now says, "but it is nonetheless true: you are what you eat—literally."

Coincidentally, Karl met a doctor practicing in a Pittsburgh suburb who held similar views about arthritis. Here and there around the country there are such doctors who, although they may not necessarily make any claims, do make a serious and conscientious effort to give as much help as possible to their arthritic patients. They tend to consider that arthritis results from a metabolic malfunction that can be corrected, and that if it is corrected in time, the healthy metabolism resulting will cure itself. What is more, some of these doctors have patients who will tell you in all sincerity that they were cured of arthritic conditions, and a few of them even have hundreds of case histories of cured patients.

Karl and the doctor worked together to develop an "anti-arthritis" diet for Karl. For years now, Karl hasn't a single trace of arthritis.

But more than 40 million Americans, more than

one out of every three adults, do have the kind of arthritis Karl suffered with—osteoarthritis. It is a disease that comes with advancing age, and 97 per cent of all people over 60 show signs of it. The Arthritis Foundation defines it as "a disease of the joints that involves a breakdown of cartilage and other tissues which make a movable joint operate properly. The damage from osteoarthritis is confined to the joints and surrounding tissues." There is good reason to believe that the breakdown in the cartilage occurs because it simply wears away through years of use. The cartilage acts as a cushion which absorbs the friction of the rubbing joints, and although it is replaced and builds up continually, in old age the building-up process seems to slacken.

When compared to rheumatoid arthritis, osteoarthritis is not a very serious disease. Although it is sometimes accompanied by pain, often it is not. But it does cripple.

The first sign of the disease is a change in the structure of the cartilage. It becomes soft, pitted and may fray. It loses its elasticity. In time, whole sections of the cartilage may be worn away, and the smooth bone ends will scrape each other. (Sometimes this scraping is actually audible.)

"As cartilage disintegrates, the joint begins to lose its normal shape, the underlying bone ends become thickened and bony spurs may form where the ligaments and capsule are attached," explains the Arthritis Foundation. "Cysts may form in the bone near the joint and fragments of bone or cartilage can become loose within the joint.

"In very severe osteoarthritis, the normal shape and mechanical structure of the joint may be destroyed."

Osteoarthritis can occur in any joint of the body, but is almost always restricted to those joints which carry weight—the hips, knees and spine. Sometimes the fingers, too, are afflicted.

What has puzzled investigators for a long time is that some few people never seem to get the disease. One theory is that their joints have developed perfectly, with no rough edges to encourage the cartilage cushions to wear out sooner. Another is that the cartilage itself may be of such high quality that it can sustain abuse beyond normal.

The traditional treatment offered by orthodox medicine is rest for the affected joints, relief of any stresses—such as from overweight or poor posture—braces or splints, hot baths, towels or heat lamps and massage. Drugs are also sometimes recommended.

None of this is particularly effective. And the one mode of treatment which men like Karl Lutz have found effective—diet therapy—has been totally avoided by orthodox medicine. An official American Medical Association statement in the February, 1968, issue of *Today's Health,* gave eight suggestions for lessening your chances of getting arthritis. They included avoiding the following: (1)

Physical stress and strain, (2) excessive fatigue, (3) over-exposure to dampness and cold, (4) joint injuries, and (5) neglect of chronic infections. Warnings were given to watch (1) overweight, (2) poor posture, and (3) occupational stress.

Although many, many researchers have stressed its importance, not one word was said about maintaining an adequate diet! Medical literature is full of references to diet in arthritis therapy. Yet, the public is unaware of those professional reports. They have been played down and hushed up by the run-of-the-mill investigators because they *are* unorthodox. They are not complicated and mystical answers, but often logical and inexpensive. They do not glorify the currently much-esteemed hypodermic needle or gelatin capsule, but rather emphasize a balanced diet and adequate nutrition.

As we have already said, arthritis is basically a disease that results from degeneration of the cartilage that lines the joints. The Arthritis and Rheumatism Foundation in discussing osteoarthritis says: "It is an incurable disease in the sense that the basic damage, which is destruction of cartilage, is practically beyond repair."

It therefore becomes clear that in considering the cause of osteoarthritis we must look chiefly for the factors that are needed for health of the cartilage of the joints.

At the outset it must be recognized that collagen, the general name for all the body's connective tissue, of which cartilage is one, is a protein tissue, since it is made up of 97.6% protein.

Probably the best and most authoritative report on collagen was made by Dr. Jerome Gross, of the Harvard Medical School, in the *Scientific American* of May, 1961. After exploring with the electron microscope and other modern research tools the process by which collagen is formed, he said: "Collagen is perhaps the most abundant protein in the animal kingdom. It is the major fibrous constituent of skin, tendon, ligament, cartilage and bone. Its properties are diverse and remarkable.

"It also underlies the development of crippling deformities associated with the rheumatic diseases and with a number of congenital defects of the skeleton, blood vessels and other connective tissue."

Since collagen is a protein tissue, primary emphasis must be placed on establishing good protein intake and assimilation.

Most people do not eat enough good protein. In a 1959 publication the Food and Nutrition Board of the National Academy of Sciences said: "Whether because of food preferences, notions about food needs, or other reasons, diets of many individuals provide less than recommended amounts of protein."

Since that was written nutritional research has placed even greater emphasis on the need for the highest quality proteins, such as eggs and the glandular meats.

Not only is there a deficiency of protein in the diets of many people, but even this inadequate amount is not properly assimilated by most older persons. This is due primarily to the fact that the secretion of hydrochloric acid in the stomach usually decreases after the age of 20. Hydrochloric acid is essential for the digestion of protein, and there is some evidence that the diminution of this acid in the stomach is due to prolonged vitamin deficiencies.

The above facts make it clear that an improvement of protein metabolism is basic in the prevention and treatment of arthritis.

Numerous references in the literature point to the fact that vitamin C is also essential for the formation and repair of collagen. These are summarized in *The Vitamins in Medicine*, Bicknell and Prescott, p. 405, *et seq.* These authors point out that while the exact mode of action is not known, it has been established that vitamin C is "directly implicated in the activity of the adrenal cortex" and that the effect of vitamin C may be to stimulate secretion of cortisone and other products of the adrenal glands (p. 406). They infer that this naturally-secreted cortisone may be essential for healthy collagen.

Another aspect of vitamin C that is important in arthritis is its primary role in maintaining elasticity of the capillaries. When vitamin C is deficient, the capillary walls readily break down and blood flows into surrounding tissues. These tiny hemorrhages tend to occur in the joints and contribute to the pain of arthritis.

All of these facts lead to the conclusion that vitamin C is of importance in connection with arthritis.

As in the case of protein, the average diet does not furnish an adequate amount of vitamin C, and special measures must be taken to supply it.

A further important fact is that vitamin C is destroyed by certain antagonists of this vitamin. One of the important functions of vitamin C is to detoxify poisons that gain access to the body. In the course of the process of neutralizing the poison, the vitamin C is destroyed. Some of these antagonists that destroy vitamin C include coffee, tobacco, and residues of pesticides that are found in most foodstuffs on the market.

It was demonstrated many years ago (in 1943) that vitamin C and calcium interact in forming collagen. In the article "Interrelation of Calcium and Ascorbic Acid," (Physiological Review, XXIII, 76) Mary E. Reid showed that adequate calcium must be present along with vitamin C and protein. A lack of calcium, or a defect of calcium metabolism may permit the collagen to degenerate.

There is good reason to believe that calcium deficiency is as prevalent as arthritis itself. Professor Roger J. Williams, says: "The position of calcium from the standpoint of its importance in nutrition and the likelihood that diets may be deficient in it, is regarded as probably unequalled by any other element." (*Biochemical Individuality,* p. 136).

Not only are average diets low in calcium, but

the many factors necessary for good utilization of calcium are not usually present.

A deficiency of almost any one of the vitamins can interfere with proper utilization of calcium. This definitely includes vitamins A, B complex, C, D, and F (essential fatty acids).

In addition, the proper acidity must be maintained in certain parts of the digestive tract.

Some of the more complex calcium compounds are utilized only if enough hydrochloric acid is present in the stomach to break them down. The small intestine should also be acid to prevent the formation of insoluble calcium compounds. The absorption of calcium is decreased by anything that stimulates the flow of alkaline digestive juices. This includes concentrated sugars and starches, such as candy, bread, etc.

When calcium is deposited out of the bloodstream in joints and other tissues, this is not necessarily a sign of excess calcium, but an indication of some defect of calcium utilization.

These are some of the many facts about calcium that must be taken into account when considering the relation of calcium deficiency to arthritis.

There is some evidence also that unsaturated fats are needed for the best health of the collagen tissues. In 1957 Dr. Hugh Sinclair of the Laboratory of Human Nutrition, University of Oxford, wrote an article entitled "Essential Fatty Acid Lack Causes Degenerative Diseases." In it Dr. Sinclair said that the essential fatty acids (abundant in certain vegetable oils and other foods) are needed for strong connective tissue. In discussing particular diseases he said:

"The so-called collagen diseases are found in highly civilized countries. . . . Such diseases include bronchial asthma, rheumatoid arthritis, certain skin diseases, and those which in general respond to cortisone."

Generally, the foods which contain unsaturated fats (good vegetable oils, fish, etc.) should be substituted for the saturated fats (animal fats, and other fats that are solid at room temperature).

Vitamin E is also important. *Chemical Week* for July 21, 1956, reported that a new theory on osteoarthritis may herald important advances against the disease. Dr. Esther Tuttle, a New York physician, told the British Commonwealth Medical Congress that osteoarthritis is not simple wear and tear on the joint, as had long been thought. Rather, she said, it is brought about by an impaired mechanism that upsets the normal balance inside the body cell. It starts with a deficiency of oxygen in the cell and then goes on to destroy the cell.

The oxygen content of the cell is of course controlled by diet. Vitamin E is the most helpful element in food for assuring the cell of enough oxygen. It works in an indirect way—by making the cell need less oxygen than it did before. Are you getting enough vitamin E to keep all your cells well oxygenated? It's been largely removed from processed foods, remember, and it is not likely that you will get enough of it unless you take supplements rich in this particular vitamin.

Actually, dietary treatment of arthritis is not a simple thing. Those few doctors who have developed it into a virtual science go about it this way:

The first step is always the same, a blood test. The test itself is routine, and is used by a great many doctors in this country. According to one authority, the American Medical Association House of Delegates reported in 1961 that blood tests of this type are among the finest diagnostic methods in existence today. United Medical Laboratories in Portland, Oregon, which is a leader in this kind of test, performs some 3 million daily.

Most doctors use a chart which contains a column showing the norm for each substance being analyzed. In every case, a significant deviation from that norm indicates the presence of certain unhealthy conditions.

The blood test is very important, since everyone has what Roger Williams of the University of Texas calls "biochemical individuality." That means that there is a world of difference between you and, say, your brother or sister. You may need twice the quantity of one nutrient, yet less than half the quantity of another, compared with your relatives. This is not theory, it is fact. No one can set a maximum or minimum daily requirement of any nutrient. To do so is to thoroughly ignore the principle of biochemical individuality.

The only sure way to tell if you are getting adequate nutrition for *you* is to take the blood test. Any deficiencies will be obvious then. If a particular case of arthritis happens to be caused by such a deficiency, it can then be effectively treated.

One such case was that of Mrs. Lucile Williams. She came to her doctor's office in a wheelchair all the way from Sacramento, California. The woman was almost paralyzed, almost totally incapacitated. After the blood test she was put on nutritional therapy. Today she is not perfect, but she is up and walking around, doing the dishes and taking care of her own home.

Another patient of the same doctor, a man, suffered from an inflexible, hypertrophic spine. Under nutritional treatment, the man can now carry on a normal day's work.

As we have already suggested, one of the biggest single factors related to arthritis is a lack of stomach acidity. Hydrochloric acid production reaches its maximum level at the age of 20 to 25. At 40, the acid has already been depleted by 15 per cent, and by the time an individual reaches 85, he has lost about 85 per cent of his stomach acidity. The problem is enhanced by alkaline drugs taken to reduce pain which people mistakenly consider acid indigestion. Alkaline foods also add to the problem.

One result is that, especially among older people, proteins go through the system largely undigested. But the human body is such that, at any cost, it will keep the blood supply of protein constant and adequate. If the protein does not come from the food, the body will draw it out of the tissues. If the protein is taken from the bursas, the collagen will break down and bursitis will develop. If from the tendons, tendosynovitis will result. If from the joints, arthritis; if from the muscles, rheumatism.

The water supply in most of our major cities hasn't helped the situation any. For example, the pH (the degree of acidity or alkalinity) of Pittsburgh drinking water, which should be around 7, was 8.2 (very alkaline) a few years ago, and it's now 8.8. The officials pour alkalies into the reservoir to reduce dirt and bacteria. But these same alkalies enhance the likelihood of painful arthritis.

To meet these problems, some doctors are giving a wide variety of dietary recommendations. First comes additional *protein*, needed to produce healthy cells—and that includes the cells which make up collagen. When there is a deficiency in protein, all the cells suffer. Protein can be found in a great many foods, but is highest in eggs, glandular meats, and muscle meats. Meat should never be cooked till well-done, however, or most of the good protein will be destroyed.

Protein foods should not be eaten with starchy ones such as bread, potatoes, corn or lima beans, however. The reason is that high-starch foods are digested much more rapidly than proteins, which take a long time to digest. Yet, the starches pull the proteins through the system rapidly, so that the proteins fail to digest. Thus, even a meal high in protein can often be of little benefit to the one eating it.

A second major aspect of the diet has to do with *carbohydrates.* Avoid all sugars, these doctors urge. The only sweetening permitted is a limited amount of honey. They also steer clear of high-starch foods such as bread and potatoes, as well as citrus fruits. According to them, they produce an alkaline residue in the stomach. Since hydrochloric acid is needed in the digestive track to break down proteins, an alkaline condition can be a precursor to arthritis.

We are merely skimming the surface here to show that diet is important—perhaps the most important single factor in controlling rheumatic disease. Yet, the establishment not only avoids it, but sometimes actually attacks the role of nutrition in arthritis therapy.

Not that poor diet is by any means the only cause of arthritis. According to Paul Tournier, M.D., there are a multitude of causes. Among those he has named in his book, *The Healing of Persons,* are: overuse of alcohol, and other manifestations of gluttony, as well as overwork and lack of exercise. Hereditary factors, reflecting wrong living in previous generations, also enter the picture, Dr. Tournier believes.

But morale conflicts have great importance as well. Many patients have been cured of arthritis when freed from fear, worry, and resentment.

"Since I first began looking systematically for morale factors in arthritis," he says, "I have not met a single case in which their importance did not at once suggest itself."

Another cause of arthritis is a physical trauma, an injury which affects the joint. Even a vaccination can be sufficient to produce the disease. Development of a case of arthritis is tied to inoculation for smallpox in a recent report in the *Archives of Internal Medicine*. Dr. Howard Silby of Buffalo, New York, reports that a 65-year-old woman was hospitalized for a 102 degree fever and a painful, swollen and stiff right knee 12 days after she had been vaccinated for smallpox. Arthritis was diagnosed. When a sample of the fluid from the right knee joint was taken, vaccinia virus (smallpox vaccine virus) was found in it. Dr. Silby suggests that doctors should look for viruses whenever the cause of arthritis is unclear.

Yet another reason some people may develop arthritis is a lack of exercise. Thus, some authorities recommend walking as one of the finest preventives of arthritis. For one thing, exercise causes the adrenal glands to produce natural cortisone which can counteract some of the effects of arthritis.

And of course exercise is doubly important for folks who have arthritis and fear the deformity and stiffness that it brings. Activity keeps the joints mobile.

There is also a relationship between foot disability and osteoarthritis. Simon J. Wikler, Doctor of Chiropody, has spent many years researching this problem. In his book, *Your Feet Are Killing You,* (Frederick Fell, Inc., New York City), he makes this observation:

"The constant pulling of joint ligaments in an imbalanced foot acts as a perpetuating agent of inflammation to the edges of the joint surface, which eventually take on a lipped and irregular appearance. The pulling of tendons and larger ligaments can be so intense with imbalanced feet that bone can be pulled away from the normal outline in the form of an osteophyte (bony outgrowth). Joints in the center of the foot (which are tighter and have a smaller range of movement) are the first to show evidence of these injuries. When the metatarsal and toe joints are affected, however, complete dislocations of the toes commonly take place, thus destroying irretrievably the balance of the foot."

Wikler also has the theory that arthritis in other parts of the body can result from arthritis of the feet. In his own private practice he has found that individuals, upon being relieved of arthritis in the feet also are cured of similar ailments in the joints of the fingers and upper extremities. One patient Wikler treated had such painful arthritis in the feet that she could hardly walk. The feet were grossly deformed, and merely massaging them caused severe pain. They were swollen, deeply calloused and she had to wear steel arch supports. All her life, the girl had had pain, occasionally so severe that she was unable to walk at all.

Most treatment, even in hospitals, offered no

relief. Finally, when she came to Dr. Wikler, the illness was so severe that he insisted she immediately reduce all standing and walking up steps to a bare minimum. The arch supports were thrown out, her feet were bandaged so that movement was restricted. Callouses were cut off and a moderate program of massage and manipulation was begun. The purpose of this was to help the feet to develop great range of movement such as would be required in walking with healthy feet. The woman was given exercises designed to stretch the shortened muscles of her legs.

Little by little the girl began wearing ordinary flat shoes. Within six months she was working as a saleswoman. Her feet had achieved a considerable range of mobility and movement. Her toes were flexible, and the woman was able to walk without pain. Improvement in the feet carried with it improvement of several other ailments.

While some of these ailments were arthritic, others were emotional, caused by the constant pain and difficulty associated with every movement.

Hip problems can also be the result of problems with the feet. Dr. Wikler also claims to have helped patients suffering from backache by means of foot treatment. He gives the case of a woman with a curvature of the spine. Further examination showed the left hip joint was turned outward and was so stiff that it was impossible to rotate the limb inward.

In Dr. Wikler's words, "The patient had sprained her ankle seven years earlier and had more or less forgotten it. The ankle was still swollen, however, and the torn ligaments were still tender. It was conjectured that, because of chronic pain to the outer side of the ankle, she had habitually turned that foot outward to avoid strain. This limited the range of movements in the hip joint, and stiffening resulted. Walking in this manner with one side of her body tilted downward had in turn caused a number of the joints in the spine to become irritated. As a matter of fact her physician had diagnosed a herniated disc of the spine."

Wikler bandaged the woman's foot and leg to force the foot inward so that she would have to use the inward rotation of the hip in spite of the fact that she was used to favoring it. In only two weeks the stiffness in the hip disappeared and the whole limb rotated inward as it normally would. "Besides," says Wikler, "the formerly obvious curvature of the spine was no longer present."

Ailing feet can easily cause aches and pains in the head and neck, too. When a person has to limp, his neck bends forward and perhaps even to one side. Holding the neck in such an unnatural position for any length of time can obviously cause sprains and aches. A farmer's wife treated by Wikler actually had developed subluxations (partial dislocations) of the vertebrae in her neck which was identifiable by x-ray, and which the doctor associated with crippled feet. Wikler treated her,

her feet became more useful and less painful, and the literal "pain in her neck" disappeared.

Cases such as these and many more which Wikler and doctors like him have experienced establish rather convincingly that at least one cause of osteoarthritis is ailing feet.

The *Fitness Encyclopedia,* (Rodale Press, 1969) says, "Physical therapy and exercise may be used successfully in treating persons suffering from osteoarthritis. It may be the most valuable treatment. Muscle weakness and loss of normal joint motion are serious end results of the disease, thereby disabling the patient. The main objective of physical therapy is keeping joints flexible, maintaining strength of the muscles so that the joints retain their stability, and protecting the joints from further injury. An attempt is made to restore the maximum degree of function.

"Physical therapy treatment must be carried on continuously, since the disease is progressive. For that reason a member of the family should learn from the therapist what exercises should be done.

"The key idea in the exercise is to see that the joints are moved through the entire range of motion, several times daily. It is extremely important, because if one joint has restricted movement, another part of the body may be affected. For example, if one hip joint is stiff the patient may favor that side, thereby weakening the muscles of the affected side and overdeveloping the muscles of the other side. Posture is affected and abnormal stresses are placed on various parts of the body, increasing the possibility of developing osteoarthritis in joints experiencing the stress.

"The exercises selected are gentle rather than vigorous. Some of these are active, done alone by the patient; other exercises are passive, in which he is assisted. The active exercises primarily develop the musculature, while the passive are directed more toward the range of motion.

"Several weeks and months may pass by before noticeable results are seen. The exercises should not be painful; or at most only slightly so. They are most effective when complete treatment is employed.

"A person may feel that his daily activities will be sufficient to develop his musculature and maintain or increase his range of motion. But, too often, daily activities do not place the joint through the entire range of motion progressively. Some daily activities, furthermore, many be violent and sharp, thereby placing strain on the osteoarthritic joints. The doctor may prescribe some daily activities, however, that he feels will not cause pain but will add to the muscle development and the range of motion.

"It is extremely important to realize that if range of motion exercises are being performed the exercises should not be forced. The movement should be gradual and progressive. That is, attempts should be made to extend the present range of motion. But pain should be kept at a minimum."

Another therapy receiving more and more attention was discussed in an article in the *New York World Telegram* for October 15, 1958. Says Horace Markley of Allandale, New Jersey, "I learned that *hot water is the oldest* curative agent in the world and that rich moderns go to hot springs to get rid of waste in their joints. The faucets were my hot springs, the washbowl and bathtub my clinic. Seated on a high stool and with a bath thermometer to tell the temperature, I plunged my hands in hot water and kept them there, then in and out of the water if it was too hot to be endured . . . I massaged and manipulated the fingers under water, flexed and pressed the knuckles. . . . Later I used a hand exerciser from a sports shop." After his hands were strong, Mr. Markley went through the same routine in the bathtub, letting the hot water "thaw" the joints of his legs.

Again it should be stressed that these methods will not be effective for everyone. In some cases, none of the methods given in this chapter will work.

Our basic point, however, is that even if your doctor has exhausted all medical techniques and given you up, you do not have to give up hoping and trying to help yourself. You know your own way of life better than anyone else. Try to analyze its own weaknesses and deficiencies, and correct them. You could find your arthritis improving beyond your expectations.

CHAPTER IV

Rheumatoid Arthritis

OF ALL THE arthritic diseases, rheumatoid arthritis is undoubtedly the most severe—both in the pain it inflicts and in the permanent crippling it causes. Victims may suffer fever, weight loss, inflammation of connective tissues and joints, swelling of the joints, excruciating pain and, in more serious cases, skeletal deformity and crippling.

More than four million Americans suffer from this systemic disease in varying stages. Most of them begin to develop rheumatoid arthritis in the prime of their lives, between the ages of 25 and 50. Usually they are between 35 and 40 when they first develop symptoms. But even children frequently fall victim to this rheumatic disease—and three women develop it for every man who does.

The first signs occur in the small joints of the hands, wrists, elbows, knees, ankles or feet. At first there will only be slight swelling of the joints—along with pain, of course. Then, suddenly and rapidly, other joints will be affected in various parts of the body.

What is actually taking place during this time is that the connective tissue in and around the joints is deteriorating. Between all joints is a lubricating substance called synovial fluid. The fluid is contained in a membrane, the synovial membrane. When rheumatoid arthritis sets in, that membrane becomes infected and inflamed. Edema, congestion, and infiltration of blood and lymph cells through the membrane can occur. The normally thin and flexible synovial membrane thickens and hardens. The process that then develops is described in the "Primer on Rheumatic Diseases":

"The synovial membrane is initially thickened by edema and cellular infiltration. Later, the membrane is thrown into folds; . . . proliferative granulomatous infiltration further thickens the synovium and capsular tissues. As the process progresses, the synovial tissue grows from the margins of the joints onto the surface of the articular cartilage or erodes between it and bone; this carpet of tissue spreading over the cartilage is referred to as pannus. The cartilage becomes eroded presumably by enzymes derived from the synovial cells or infiltrating leukocytes or both. The subchondral bone can also be eroded by invading pannus, and granulation tissue in the marrow spaces beneath the articular cortex can form fibrotic cysts. The bones in the vicinity of diseased joints become osteoporotic. Erosion of the articular cartilage and bone can progress to total destruction of the original joint surfaces. Adhesions between opposing layers of pannus can lead to fibrous ankylosis of the joint. The fibrous tissue may ultimately be replaced by bone, completely obliterating the original joint."

But all this talk about synovial membranes and joints ought not to give the impression that rheumatoid arthritis is restricted to these areas. Unlike osteoarthritis, rheumatoid arthritis is a disease which can affect the whole body—it is what scientists call a systemic illness. It may involve the heart, nerves, muscles, and other tissues and organs.

The $64,000 question, of course, is what causes rheumatoid arthritis? To answer that question would be to fling wide the doors of potential treatments, cures and even prevention. But the hard fact is that the causes of arthritis are just not known in most cases.

We speak of "causes" and not "cause" because one thing that *is* known is that rheumatoid arthritis does not have a single cause. It might be compared to a sprained ankle. Many factors can cause the sprain, although there is only one kind of symptom.

One of the causes of rheumatoid arthritis—at

least in theory—is infection. That idea has been receiving a considerable amount of attention lately. A group of Edinburgh, England, doctors and research workers have isolated diphtheroid bacteria from the joints of arthritics. They said in 1966, "We believe that the presence of these bacteria within cells of the linings of the joint (the synovial membrane) may cause the defense mechanism to react against these cells, causing chronic inflammation.

"If this idea is correct," they said, "the presence of these bacteria may prove to be of fundamental importance in the causation of the disease and may profoundly influence its future treatment."

Another who holds to the infection theory is Dr. Ephraim P. Engleman, clinical professor of medicine at the University of California, whose research has implicated an infectious organism common among animals and also found in the joints of afflicted patients and which, injected into the knee joints of monkeys, produced arthritis.

Various infections have been known to cause arthritis, but none that has been isolated would produce the rheumatoid type. Infectious organisms have been implicated because they interfere with the chemical processes in the joints and the result is the characteristic swelling, inflammation and disintegration of protective tissue between the bones. Dr. Engleman told a seminar for science writers sponsored by the Arthritis Foundation and the University of Chicago (*Chicago Tribune*, May 9,

1967), that the suspected organism lives in cells, and is commonly found in cattle, hogs, sheep, mice and other animals. When it infects humans, it ordinarily causes inflammation of the eyes and the urethra in addition to arthritis.

In spite of the circumstantial evidence implicating viruses, proof of the connection has been evasive in rheumatoid arthritis. It may be that such evidence will never, in fact, be found.

Hormonal imbalance has also been considered responsible for certain cases of rheumatoid arthritis. Again, however, conclusive evidence is lacking.

There is good reason to suspect, though, that one's dietary status can be directly associated with rheumatoid arthritis. For example, using 31 patients and giving them four grams of unsaturated fatty acids daily along with a general vitamin supplement for three months, Dr. Worne, M.D., and Dr. Schneider, Ph.D., found and reported in the August, 1954 *Archives of Research* that the fatty acids are "of major importance as adjuncts in the treatment of rheumatoid arthritis." They admitted that they do not know why. But they presented a theory having to do with intricate chemical changes that go on in the body which they think may explain the results they got.

Before starting their treatment they tested the blood of the patients for vitamin C and the fatty acids. Before the treatment began the levels of these two important food elements ranged from .30 to .80 milligrams per cubic centimeter for vitamin C and 108 to 183 for the unsaturated fatty acids. At the end of the experiment the blood was tested again and the range was from .63 to 1.30 for vitamin C and from 171 to 329 for the fats. Quite a difference! We do not know why the vitamin C level was checked in this instance, nor do the authors mention what part vitamin C may have played in this story.

What were the exact results of the treatment described above? The three cases of children involved were completely cured. Their blood chemistries were normal, joint swelling and all tenderness and swelling were eliminated and all gained weight and were able to return to normal activity. The rest of the cases, with the exception of four, were classified as completely relieved as far as arthritis symptoms were concerned. They, too, returned to their usual activities.

It is unfortunate that these researchers did not appraise the role of vitamin C in obtaining these results. But other researchers have investigated the vitamin and its relationship to arthritis. One such researcher is W. J. McCormick, M.D. of Toronto. He described his findings in an article, "The Rheumatic Diseases," in the *Archives of Pediatrics* for April, 1955. Dr. McCormick tells us that only recently have we classified these diseases according to the way they manifest themselves—rheumatic fever, rheumatoid arthritis, primary osteoarthritis, rheumatoid spondylitis, bursitis, synovitis and so forth. The one thing all these diseases appear to have in common, says he, is that the cartilages involved in joints and the connective tissue surrounding them disintegrate. So it seems that, if one could explain this one symptom, one could get to the bottom of the matter.

Dr. McCormick believes that the early writers on scurvy gave the most significant clues to the cause and cure of arthritis. Scurvy? How is it possible? Scurvy is a disease of long ago, before we knew the value of fresh raw foods in the diet. Nobody in our enlightened era ever has scurvy! Or do they? Listen to Dr. McCormick's reasoning and make up your own mind.

He quotes James Lind, who wrote medical treatises in 1753, as saying that in scurvy the muscles are so lax and tender that they readily fall apart during autopsies. He said, too, that scurvy affected the cartilage of the ribs so decidedly as to sometimes separate them entirely from the breast bone. He had no explanation for the fact that "scurvy seats itself so commonly in the joint of the knee."

Lind reviewed the findings of earlier writers on scurvy who had observed that the bones of the scurvy patient cracked when he moved. "In some we perceived a small low noise when they breathed. . . . The ligaments of the joints were corded and loose. Instead of finding in the cavities of the joints the usual sweet oily mucilage there was only a greenish liquor . . . gout is known to proceed from scurvy."

It is well to remember that two or three hundred years ago medical students had ample opportunity to study scurvy. It was nearly as common as colds are today. So, from many autopsies, they knew the symptoms of this disease, then so puzzling, which as we know today, is the result of a deficiency in vitamin C.

"The most definitely established function of vitamin C is that of assisting in the formation of collagen for the maintenance of integrity and stability of the connective tissues generally, and this would include the bones, cartilages, muscles and vascular tissues," says Dr. McCormick. Collagen is the substance that is so important in all connective tissue—the material that makes gelatin when you boil bones and cartilages. "In a deficiency of this vitamin (C)," Dr. McCormick continues, "instability and fragility of all such tissues is believed to be caused by the breakdown of intercellular cement substance, resulting in easy rupture of any and all of these connective tissues" which would include the discs of the backbone, the ligaments and small sacs in the interior of the joints, and the cartilage which helps in the movement of joints. The vulnerability of these joints may be, then, the common cause for the rheumatic diseases, says Dr. McCormick.

Coming up to modern times, we find two researchers, Rinehart and Mettier, who correlated deficiency of vitamin C with rheumatic disease. In an article in *The American Journal of Pathology,* vol. 10, page 61, 1934, they relate that they found impairment of the joints in animals deprived of vitamin C. When the animals were subject to some infection, the joint symptoms became worse. Those animals which were subjected to the same infection while on a diet rich in vitamin C did not develop the joint disorders.

Extending these researches further, Rinehart found that the amount of vitamin C in the blood of arthritic and rheumatic fever patients is extremely low. He believes that the important basic cause of rheumatic disease is infection, superimposed on a vitamin C deficiency. Dr. McCormick believes that both the infection and the rheumatism are direct results of vitamin C deficiency.

In this article, we find reference to many different examples—a mouth infection associated with rheumatic fever which was shown to be due to vitamin C deficiency; a streptococcus and pneumonia epidemic in a naval training school which did not affect students who were taking liberal doses of vitamin C; a report on a less-than-usual excretion of vitamin C in rheumatoid arthritis patients who were getting plenty of the vitamin in their diets—seeming to indicate that the vitamin was being used at a faster than normal rate.

Rinehart, in a paper read before the California Heart Association, May 6, 1944, told of his findings that vitamin P (the flavonoids) used in conjunction with vitamin C had a favorable influence on the condition of the blood vessels in infections. It seems to us that Rinehart may have the answer right here—that is, that natural vitamin C, which occurs along with vitamin P in foods, may be what the rheumatic tissues lack—not just vitamin C as it appears in synthetic preparations, unaccompanied by any of the other food elements.

Dr. McCormick, a great believer in the use of vitamins for prevention and for cure, tells us that he has given massive doses of vitamin C in injections and orally in a number of cases of rheumatic fever. "The patients made rapid and complete recovery in three or four weeks without cardiac complication." The usual hospital treatment may go on for three or four months, with cortisone or aspirin being given and a high rate of heart complications. Dr. McCormick has also given massive doses of vitamin C in cases of "incipient arthritis" —that is, arthritis which is just beginning, with "similarly favorable results."

What does he mean by "massive doses?" From one to 10 grams daily. That is, in terms in which one buys vitamin C products—from 1,000 milligrams to 10,000 milligrams a day. Is it necessary for the average person on an average diet to take this much vitamin C in order to prevent arthritis? We believe not. These are curative doses for patients who already have the symptoms of disease. However, we do not think it is possible to get too much vitamin C in your diet these days and it is likely that most of us are getting far too little.

How does this happen in an age when fresh vegetables and fresh fruits are available the year round? Too many other foods are available too—worthless foods—soft drinks, pastries, candies, cakes, etc. Every mouthful of these foods that your family eats means that they can eat less of fresh foods. Just in the case of children, how much of their diet consists of worthless foods compared to their daily intake of fresh raw foods?

An article from the *Journal of the American Dietetic Association* for May, 1954, gives us part of the answer. In a survey of 131 children with rheumatic fever, compared with 131 carefully paired children who did not have the disease, it was found that the rheumatic fever children were eating less of vitamin C-rich foods than the healthy children. The sick children did not get even one serving per day of foods that contain even moderate amounts of vitamin C.

In another survey it was found on autopsies of infants dying at Johns Hopkins that 6 per cent of them suffered from scurvy. In still another survey reported in the *Journal of the American Dietetic Association* it was shown that of a group of school children studied, 47 per cent had a low intake of vitamin C, and 53 per cent had a low blood level of the vitamin. College students eating at dining halls were found to be eating meals 62 per cent of which were deficient in vitamin C.

In another survey of institutional inmates over the age of 50, it was found that 87 per cent *were deficient in vitamin C*. Dr. McCormick tells us that he has examined more than 500 patients with particular reference to their vitamin C status and has found that less than 10 per cent of them have had the optimum amount of vitamin C in their blood at any time.

Remember, too, that vitamin C is most perishable, so that even today with our wonderful methods of transportation and marketing the fruits and vegetables you buy may have lost much of their vitamin C by the time you buy them. Storing and cooking destroy much more of it. The poisonous substances to which you are exposed day after day use it up. Cigarette smoke is an enemy of vitamin C in your tissues, for example.

If, indeed, lack of vitamin C is responsible for initiating rheumatic troubles of all kinds, is it any wonder that the medical journals report dolefully that practically everybody over the age of forty has or shortly will have arthritic symptoms?

An article in *Clinical Medicine,* volume 52, page 157, 1945, stressed the importance of treating arthritis with vitamin C, along with a related nutrient, vitamin D.

In another report, four researchers studied 42 patients with rheumatoid arthritis and 17 patients with osteoarthritis over a period of seven years to discover how their health could be improved if they took quite large doses of these two vitamins every day. The story of their findings as reported in *The Journal of American Geriatrics* for June, 1956, is amazing. The authors are Peter J. Warter, M.D. of McKinley Hospital, Trenton, N.J., Dominic A.

Donio, M.D., of Sacred Heart Hospital, Allentown, Pa., and Steven Horoschak, B.S. of the National Drug Company.

The authors remind us that all of us are troubled with minor injuries during every day. We bump our ankles, pinch our fingers, stumble over cracks in the sidewalk, hit our heads on the cellar stairs and so on. Usually we pay no attention to these knocks except for a casual "Oh, I wonder where I got that bruise." "That bruise" means that capillaries have hemorrhaged. You are bleeding internally, even if ever so slightly. Our authors tell us that these bleedings might well develop into something serious in a defective capillary system, made so by poisons of various kinds—drugs, for instance, or tobacco.

Furthermore, they tell us that rheumatic fever is believed to be a disease of the blood vessels, involving fragility of these small capillaries so that they burst easily. High blood pressure or hypertension is another disease in which the stability of the capillaries is of utmost importance. Patients who have fragile capillaries often have strokes, hemorrhages in the retina of the eye and other serious disorders. So it seems certain that disorders of the capillary system are at the bottom of many chronic diseases.

What are the capillaries made of? Cells and intercellular material. We know positively that the intercellular material is kept in repair by vitamin C. We know that in scurvy, the disease of vitamin

C deficiency, there is a breakdown of this intercellular material which can be reversed almost magically by giving vitamin C. Walter H. Eddy in his book *What are the Vitamins?* (Reinhold, 1941) says he thinks that "country rheumatism" which develops at the end of a long winter is nothing more or less than hemorrhaging capillaries in the joints, as a result of vitamin C deficiency.

Later researchers have shown that vitamin C cannot function well in the absence of vitamin P or the bioflavonoids, as they are sometimes called. Then, too, vitamin P does not take its part in body processes without vitamin C being present. So, in testing the effect of vitamin C on arthritic patients, the authors felt it necessary to add vitamin P as well.

They tested the rheumatoid arthritis patients for capillary fragility and found that it was almost universal. In other words, pressure on the capillaries caused them to burst. These folks consistently have bruised themselves from everyday bumps. Blood pressure was low in these patients; the heart beat was rapid. The 17 osteoarthritis patients were obese and had high blood pressure. In the most severe cases of the rheumatoid arthritis patients, as much as 600 to 1,000 milligrams of vitamin P-vitamin C (in equal amounts) were given daily in divided doses. Gradually the dose was reduced to 300 milligrams daily. For milder cases 400 to 600 milligrams were given at the beginning, and these were then reduced to 300 for a "maintenance dose." In the osteoarthritic patients, the treatment was begun and maintained with 300 milligram doses. The reason given for the larger doses in rheumatoid arthritis is that there is inflammation in this disease which taxes the capillary resistance to a greater degree.

What were the results obtained? In the rheumatoid group, normal capillary resistance was established in 6 to 8 weeks. That means no more bruises for them. These patients apparently utilized their food better too, for protein and vitamin B supplements brought a gain in weight and an increase in red blood, to combat anemia. This did not happen in patients who were not taking the vitamins. The blood pressure in most patients soon came to normal range. Some of the patients who had been subject to colds voluntarily reported that they had much more resistance to cold, even though the researchers were not testing for this angle. The arthritis, which improved steadily, flared up again when the vitamins were discontinued for several months in the case of a few patients. There were no strokes or other blood vessel disorders.

In the osteoarthritic group, those who bruised easily developed resistance to bruising within 6 weeks. Six patients with high blood pressure brought their pressure down to normal. The authors admit that rest and diet may have played some part in this, but they believe the vitamins should get some credit. The arthritic symptoms improved. Even though damage to joints could not, of course, be repaired, the patients had less fatigue, less discomfort in the joints and general improvement.

The conclusions of the authors are that the combination of vitamin P and vitamin C has the capacity to correct abnormal capillary fragility and permeability and thus enhances the effectiveness of therapy directed against the rheumatic diseases.

The only way to get all of the elements—both vitamin P and vitamin C—is to eat foods that contain them all and to take natural food supplements rich in them all. The foods you should be sure to get in ample quantity are mostly raw fruits. Grapes, plums, black currants, apricots, cherries and blackberries are good sources of vitamin P. And the citrus fruits. Other foods rich in vitamin C are broccoli, brussels sprouts, cabbage, dandelion greens, melons, cantaloupes, tomatoes, mustard greens, green peppers.

Vitamin D alone for arthritis seems to be a treatment that carries little if any risk and one which can be applied with a good chance of success as a preventive measure.

We found recently in a 1935 medical journal the account of the treatment of a number of patients with vitamin D. Two physicians, Dr. Irving Dreyer and Dr. C. I. Reed of the University of Illinois Department of Medicine, writing in the *Archives of Physical Therapy,* volume 16, page 537, 1935, have this to say, "In general, the results suggest that this material may prove an efficient form of therapy as well as a valuable aid in the study of the fundamental nature of arthritis."

They treated 67 patients, who were suffering from a variety of arthritic afflictions. Forty-four of these showed clinical improvement, 13 showed none and 10 cases were uncertain. About 200 other cases being treated privately showed approximately the same results. The doctors gave massive doses of synthetic vitamin D.

Since vitamin D is one of the two vitamins (vitamin A is the other) which has been known to produce toxic results if taken in too large a dosage over a long period of time, it is interesting to know that these arthritic patients were started on a daily dosage of 200,000 units of synthetic vitamin D. This dosage was given daily for a month. If there was no improvement and no indication that any harm had been done by this quite large dose, it was increased by 50,000 to 60,000 units each week until there was some improvement or indication of overdosage. In some stubborn cases it was found necessary to increase to 600,000 units or even to 1,000,000 for a few days and then reduce again to 200,000. "Most of our results have been obtained with daily doses of 300,000 to 500,000 units," say the authors.

They tell us that they do not believe vitamin D in such enormous doses poses any greater risk than many preparations used daily by physicians. And, they say, one knows within a few weeks if symptoms of overdosage are present. When the vitamin is discontinued, the symptoms disappear.

It is interesting, too, to note that some patients who could not take massive doses of vitamin D found that they could manage perfectly well if large doses of brewer's yeast were given at the same time. This is not successful in every case, they say, but they tell us of one woman patient who, on 3 successive occasions, with intervals of 2 to 3 weeks between, took 300,000 units daily for 10 days, but became nauseated on the 11th day. Nausea is one of the first symptoms that too much vitamin D is being taken. When she took 6 grams of brewer's yeast three times daily she was able to take up to 600,000 units of vitamin D daily for 3 weeks without becoming nauseated, or suffering from other unpleasant symptoms.

"The total number of human subjects to whom large doses of viosterol (synthetic vitamin D) have been administered for all conditions now numbers approximately 700," say our authors. They continue, "Of these, 63 have, at some time, manifested evidence of toxicity. The actual size of the dose producing toxicity varies in different individuals. Human subjects have received as high as 3,000,000 units daily for 5 days. Single large doses have been given by others. It is apparent, however, that toxicity is more likely to occur after prolonged administration of moderate amounts than as a result of brief administration of larger amounts."

So what lessons can we learn from the work that was reported on vitamin D for arthritis cases? It seems to us that we should learn that vitamin D is indeed essential for adults and perhaps lack of it may be a definite factor in the cause of arthritis. No one knows apparently why the vitamin brings relief in those cases where it does. Couldn't it be simply that there was a lack of the vitamin? Vitamin D is almost completely lacking in food. Our chief source of it is sunlight which, falling on our bare skin, produces a substance which the body then changes into vitamin D. Doesn't it seem quite likely that people who spend most of their time indoors could very definitely be lacking in vitamin D, especially in the winter months when the sunlight is weak and infrequent?

We had never heard before of any relationship between the taking of brewer's yeast (rich chiefly in vitamin B and minerals) and protection against the possible toxicity of large doses of vitamin D. But it seems to indicate yet another in the complex series of relationships indicating that one is safest to take whole foods and to take all the important minerals and vitamins in natural food supplements like brewer's yeast that we do not know anything about as yet. If it protects against toxicity of large doses of vitamin D, perhaps it also acts to protect us against many other unknown poisons in our environment.

We would not suggest that readers attempt to

cure arthritic conditions by using massive doses of vitamin D as the doctors at the university hospital did unless they are taking these doses under the supervision of a capable doctor who understands just what the symptoms of overdosage may be. But the fact is that ample evidence exists to indicate that vitamin D may help to control arthritis.

CHAPTER V

The Anti-Arthritis Diets

MANY RESEARCHERS have reported evidence that not only particular vitamins and nutrients but actual foods play an important part in preventing—and in some cases causing—arthritis. We will discuss some of those foods in this chapter.

Probably no food has received as much attention in arthritis prevention as has honey. But the debate on whether or not it really works is, to say the least, controversial. Two letters recently received express both sides of the controversy.

The writers were Mrs. Ida Crowther of Cass City, Michigan, and F. H. Young of Long Beach, California. Mrs. Crowther owns an apiary—that is, she raises bees. She told us that she had been suffering from a quite severe case of arthritis for months and had tried every known combination of foods in an effort to cure it. She noticed that the pain disappeared when she was helping her husband extract honey—and of course eating some honey while she worked—and appeared again when she was not working around the honey. Then one day she read in the *Bee Journal* an article on *Honey and Arthritis,* written by D. C. Jarvis, M.D., who said that honey had been used many times as a cure for arthritis. She at once began to take five tablespoons of honey per day. Within two weeks the swelling in her knee was gone. "And now a year later," says Mrs. Crowther, "I have never quit taking the honey and I can sit on the floor now with both my knees lying flat. . . . I would advise all who suffer from arthritis to turn to honey and use plenty of protein and whole milk, plenty of wheat germ and enough of brewers' yeast and a generous green salad, with an occasional fruit salad, all with lemon juice dressing and a little honey added for taste." Incidentally, Mrs. Crowther is on a reducing diet and has had no trouble in losing many pounds, even with her high-calorie honey every day.

Mr. Young's letter, in the same mail, told us just the opposite. He had noticed the beginnings of arthritis about five years ago, and changing his diet around, found that *by omitting his usual honey on his morning cereal and toast, he could cause the pain of the arthritis to disappear.* A friend had the same experience.

The article from the *Bee World* to which Mrs.

Crowther referred talks about the ratio of calcium to phosphorus in the bloodstream. We know that this ratio is important and that too much phosphorus will throw it off balance. Dr. Jarvis states that inflammation in the body is caused by a high phosphorus level, with not enough calcium to balance it. Cereals, beans and other seed-foods are high in phosphorus and many of us have far too much of this kind of food in our meals to the exclusion of calcium-containing foods. In fact it is accepted among nutritionists that most of us lack calcium.

Dr. Jarvis says that when the phosphorus level is high, the intense pain of arthritis is present. Honey raises the calcium level and lowers the phosphorus level. He says that one tablespoon of honey taken to relieve the pain will lower the phosphorus level of the blood for as long as 24 hours, after which it will return again to its original level, unless of course you take more honey.

Several questions remain in our minds. How does it happen that other foods high in calcium do not have this same effect? Why won't milk produce relief from swelling, or eggs, or any of the vegetables that are high in calcium? Or could it be possible that Mrs. Crowther's honey was superior—honey from her own hives which she knew contained no adulterant? Perhaps Mr. Young's honey contained sucrose artificially added, perhaps it contained residues of insecticides.

Dr. Jarvis and Mrs. Crowther are not the only ones to believe honey can help arthritis. There is an anti-stiffness factor in honey right from the comb, that has not been heated, according to a report made before the Federation of American Societies for Experimental Biology, and reported in the *Journal of the American Dietetic Association* for September, 1954.

Moderate wrist stiffness in guinea pigs, similar to arthritis in man, was cured in a week with a daily dose of 1/2 gram of honey or wax from the comb. That's about one-fifteenth of an ounce. More severe cases required a little longer time.

Animals treated with honey that had been boiled for thirty minutes were not helped by the treatment. One theory is that there may be a new "x" vitamin which is missing in the diets of arthritics. The most important aspect of this story, we believe, is that the honey used in the treatment is raw—just as it comes from the bees. Raw honey is one of the few foods remaining that have not been processed or meddled with in some way.

We don't have the answer to the whole problem of honey in its relation to arthritis. But, as you know, for some reason, bees have consistently been associated with arthritis cures. Bee venom, containing formic acid, is used in many parts of the world as a rheumatism cure. Honey contains an infinitesimally small amount of this acid. We'd suggest that, if you suffer from arthritis, you try the suggestion of honey with meals. But make certain you are getting pure honey, as free as possible from insecticides and make certain too that it has not been heated, clarified, or treated in any other way.

We have been discussing at some length what foods may be of help to arthritics. There are also some foods which should be avoided, according to some medical reports. For example, in *Medical World News* (Dec. 18, 1964) we read, "Cereals may be the staff of life, but some of them might also be culprits in rheumatoid arthritis, according to Dr. Raymond Shatin of the Alfred Hospital in Malvern, Australia. He links the disease to malabsorption of digested foods which he blames on a deficiency of gluten-splitting enzymes. Dr. Shatin sees evidence for the validity of his theory in the higher incidence of rheumatoid arthritis among wheat consuming people than among those who subsist largely on rice and corn meal. And he suggests that the disease can be managed by diet:

"The proposed corrective regimen consists of high-protein, gluten-free diet with vitamin supplements, antihistamines, and anabolic agents." Thus treated, arthritics in Dr. Shatin's practice who previously depended on anti-inflammatory therapy have gradually been able to give it up.

Shatin adds food supplements to his therapeutic regimen for arthritis in rheumatism.

An article in *Prevention* 10 years earlier noted that "The frequency of liver disorder in arthritics suggests that the liver might be unable to do its work of transforming carotene into vitamin A, so that a greater quantity of vitamin A would be necessary in the patient's diet. . . . Most arthritics have difficulty in assimilating carbohydrates—that is, starches and sugars. This suggests deficiency of vitamin B which is the vitamin necessary to accompany these substances on their way through the digestive tract. . . ."

Another theory is that bread—another major part of the average diet which contains gluten—may be related to arthritis. Dr. Shatin has also done research on that theory.

Other nutrients which have been reported useful in treating arthritis are the bioflavonoids. In a study conducted by James R. West of the Morrell Memorial Hospital, Lakeland, Florida, 21 patients with varying degrees of rheumatoid arthritis were given 2,000 to 3,000 milligrams of bioflavonoids daily for two to six months. Catharyn Elwood reports on the study in her book, *Feel Like a Million* (Devin-Adair, 23 East 26th Street, N.Y.).

Here is a typical case. A 52-year-old woman with rheumatoid arthritis in both hands, wrists and elbows, and in the right shoulder, knees and ankles was given 3,000 milligrams of bioflavonoid complex.

In seven days she "felt better." In two weeks the pain had practically gone, her digestion was improved and bowel action normal. Her blood pressure dropped from 190 to 176, and by the end of five weeks she had more action in her joints and more endurance than she had known in several years. This was a very severe case with crippling changes in the joints. Her improvement was described as "dramatic."

It is quite common today to hear people complain about bursitis. Doctors Biskind and Martin have secured "rapid and complete relief" with this ailment when bioflavonoids were given. For instance, one 38-year-old man with severe subpatellar (knee joint) bursitis had extensive local swelling, local heat, extreme tenderness, severe pain, and limitation of motion. With 200 milligrams of bioflavonoids three times a day—a total of 600—the swelling and pain were almost completely gone in 24 hours. In 72 hours the lesion had subsided almost completely leaving only slight local tenderness.

In Melbourne, Australia, Dr. Shatin examined thirty patients at the Alred Hospital, all suffering from the "incurable" rheumatoid arthritis, and treated them with an experimental drugless treatment that consisted entirely of controlled diet. Twenty of them had striking remissions of the disease. At the time the new treatment was reported on in the *Medical Journal of Australia* (August 1, 1964) the remissions had been maintained for substantial periods by all, in some cases for as long as 18 months.

Remember, this is rheumatoid arthritis, the agonizing inflammation of the joints that has received the attention of thousands of very fine doctors, and for which nearly every known drug has been attempted as a treatment, in the hope of stumbling on something that would bring relief. The best that has ever been done up to now has been the securing of temporary remission with the cortical steroid hormones (cortisone, ACTH, etc.) at the cost of subsequent damage to the bone. And after a few months of steroid treatment, the stiffness returns and the pain is as bad as ever. So that now, even though there are only twenty patients reported on, out of a total of 30 in the experiment, who have secured seemingly permanent remissions, this 66 per cent success by dietary means alone takes on enormous significance.

What was this astonishingly beneficial diet? Simply a high protein diet with vitamin supplements and the one added feature that all gluten was rigorously eliminated.

Gluten is the incomplete protein substance that is formed when water is added to wheat. It has a special sticky, rubbery quality that provides a perfect trap for carbon dioxide bubbles formed in the baking process, so that bread containing gluten rises and makes the high loaf with which we are all familiar. Present to a lesser extent in rye, but entering the diet of most people chiefly through wheat products, it is gluten that makes breads, cakes, and other wheat-containing foods a problem in assimilation for all too many people.

As much is indicated in the *Australian Medical Journal* report by Dr. R. Shatin, the physician who conducted the experiment. After pointing out that the cereal grains, which were introduced into man's diet comparatively late in human history, represented a radical change in diet that "confronted man's metabolism with an historic challenge," Dr. Shatin states: "The pathogenesis of rheumatoid arthritis, as put forward in this concept, rests on the inherited susceptibility . . . which can be activated by the environmental factor, gluten . . . into a primary and fundamental lesion—enteropathy."

His theory, to put it in simpler language, is that an inherited inability to metabolize gluten leads to a malfunction of the intestine (such as occurs in celiac disease) and that this in turn causes rheumatoid arthritis. It does not cause it in all people, obviously, or everyone who eats wheat or rye would be suffering from this vicious ailment. But enough people do suffer from it, their number running into the millions in the United States alone, to indicate how widespread is the intolerance to gluten, if Dr. Shatin is right.

If future researches demonstrate conclusively that he is right—it seems quite likely—then it may ultimately be found that at least a majority of cases of rheumatoid arthritis can be eliminated by eliminating gluten from the diet. Dr. Shatin does not consider this incomplete cereal protein the only responsible element. He points to other factors "such as infection, trauma or drugs acting on the small intestine." But two-thirds of his patients secured remissions on the gluten-free diet.

Of the four case histories related by Dr. Shatin, the first is that of a woman of 53 who had been anemic since adolescence. This had led to various infections, and even when the anemia was improved by treatment, there was "recurrent constipation with intermittent diarrhea." In time she developed rheumatoid arthritis in the right shoulder girdle, an ailment not only extremely painful but threatening to render this divorced woman unable to work, since she was a private secretary. She was treated with "salicylates, butazolidin, chloroquine, and short courses of synthetic corticosteroids."

"In two weeks on (gluten-free) treatment the patient improved noticeably, and gained two pounds in weight. . . . At the time of writing, two years later, her condition was better than during the whole of the ten years preceding the new treatment."

Case history number two relates to a male clerk, 62 years old, who suffered from arthritis in both shoulders, the right hip, a portion of the spine and in his hands. In six months of treatment "the use of butazolidin, antimalaria drugs, synthetic corticosteroids and a profusion of salicylates alleviated his symptoms, but the grip remained weak, walking was painful and the erythrocyte sedimentation rate increased to 60 mm. in one hour. Because of this unsatisfactory response to the recognized treatment, and the fact that the patient was faced with loss of employment, the testing of the regime based on the new concept followed. His response was dramatic—alimentary discomfort disappearing within 48 hours. Within less than a week, he was completely free from pain and able to clench both fists—a feat he had been unable to accomplish for nearly six months."

Why should the inability to digest and absorb gluten lead to the development of rheumatoid arthritis?

We can find two clues in the laboratory tests that are used to diagnose the illness. First, the Merck Manual tells us that "A moderate hypochromic, normocytic anemia not responsive to iron almost always is present during the active stages." This indicates that an active attack of rheumatoid arthritis is somehow associated with the rapid destruction of the red blood cells for a cause that is not associated with iron deficiency. This is a condition that is determined in the laboratory by the rate of erythrocyte sedimentation, which is to say the rate at which a sediment of dead cells is thrown off when blood is whirled in a special instrument.

A study on the effect of diet on the erythrocyte sedimentation rate was published in August, 1964, in the *Journal of the Alabama Medical Association,* by E. Cheraskin and W. M. Ringsdorf, Jr., the noted researchers of the University of Alabama Medical Center. Making a double-blind study on 84 male dental students, these investigators found that both abnormally high and abnormally low rates of decay of the red blood cells could be corrected in a few days' time by a diet that eliminated carbohydrate and added 40 grams a day of a high grade protein supplement. By eliminating carbohydrate from the diet, Cheraskin and Ringsdorf inevitably eliminated all gluten, which is found only in the carbohydrate foods that all the cereal grains are. And it is entirely possible that it is the elimination of the gluten, rather than the undifferentiated carbohydrate, that did the trick of bringing the rate of reproduction and death of the red blood cells to normalcy.

Why this should be so was indicated in the *AMA Journal* (May 18, 1957) in a very informative article by James B. Allison, Ph.D., of the Bureau of Biological Research and the Department of Physiology and Biochemistry of Rutgers University. Gluten, he pointed out, is a protein that is exceptionally deficient in 2 of the 10 essential amino acids —lysine and tryptophan. "If the food protein is deficient in one or more of the essential amino acids," he stated, "tissue protein synthesis will be restricted, and some of the dietary amino acids will enter catabolic pathways." Catabolic means destructive, and it is entirely possible that one of the paths of destruction taken by the uncompleted amino acids of gluten is destruction of the red blood cells.

Dr. Allison goes on to show that the ability of the liver to remove toxic wastes is sharply reduced by protein depletion, such as is brought about by feeding with low-grade protein, such as gluten. And this brings us back to Dr. Shatin's theory as described in the *Medical Journal of Australia,* and the second clue to how gluten may cause rheumatoid arthritis.

Dr. Shatin believes that in many people, selected by their own heredity, the inability of the intestine to absorb gluten leads to the establishment of antibodies. This toxicity of gluten could be because it steals sufficient protein from the liver, as believed by Dr. Allison, or it could depend on some toxic substance in the gluten itself. There are many who believe that one of the amino acid compounds of which it is made up—the one named gliadin—is the toxic agent. But in either case, that some people would react to this toxicity by the formation of antibodies is entirely plausible. And if we check the *Merck Manual* for the laboratory findings that establish rheumatoid arthritis, sure enough we find that an abnormal gamma globulin, which is to say an abnormal type of systemic antibodies, is found in 60 to 70 per cent of rheumatoid arthritis cases.

It is Dr. Shatin's concept that every time gluten is eaten, the body rushes gamma globulin to the intestine to fight it just as it would fight any infection. One result is a constantly inflamed condition of the intestine and Dr. Shatin believes that this chronic inflammation spreads out and is carried into the joints, producing the condition of rheumatoid arthritis.

Hereditary intolerance to gluten is not universal, although we believe that we have shown that gluten does nobody any good. Nevertheless, as Dr. Shatin very ably points out, there is no way that you can tell whether or not you possess this hereditary intolerance. If gluten inflames your intestine, it has probably been doing so all your life and the condition will seem perfectly normal to you—until, late in life, you find that you have rheumatoid arthritis or some other type of chronic inflammation. Why take such a chance? Even if you have no sharp toxic reaction, gluten cannot possibly do you any good. It can only rob your body of the complete proteins that are needed by every living cell.

Several basic diets have been developed for victims of arthritis. Diets for arthritics containing plenty of fat but little in the way of sweets got a nod from researchers at a meeting of the Endocrine Society in Chicago several years ago. According to *Science News Letter* for June 14, 1952, patients on such a diet showed significant improvement in their symptoms but when starch and sugar were placed in the diet, pain and other symptoms tended to return.

Another system of dieting for relief of arthritis was proposed in an article by two physicians from Cambridge, Massachusetts published in *The Journal of the National Medical Association* for July, 1959.

A summary of the article, written for inclusion in scientific books, tells us that the diet produced major clinical and hematological (blood) improvement in arthritis and rheumatism. According to the summary, the main points in this new system are the taking of cod liver oil on an empty stomach and the restriction of all water intake to a single portion taken one hour before breakfast.

The article is well written and thorough in the detail with which the authors have cared for their patients and followed through, during the six-month treatment, to check on their welfare. One hundred and forty arthritic patients were originally scheduled for the test, but some had to drop out, so final facts are given on the 98 who could follow the suggested diet that was being tested over this period.

The results were excellent. Dr. Charles A. Brusch, M.D., and Edward T. Johnson, M.D., the authors, tell us that 92 of the patients showed major improvement in their arthritic symptoms and favorable changes in their blood chemistry. The blood sedimentation rate dropped to normal. Cholesterol levels dropped or could be controlled, even though eggs, butter, milk and cod liver oil were everyday items of diet. Blood sugar levels "turned to the lower side of normal," say our authors. One diabetic patient was compelled to give up taking insulin. Blood pressure levels were found to be lower at the end of the experiment.

Doesn't all this sound just wonderful from the point of view of health? Doesn't it sound as though our authors have uncovered a veritable treasure of information and a simple-as-can-be system for guaranteeing good health to most of us, just with a few small rules about drinking water and taking cod liver oil?

But wait a moment! Although the summary of the article states just "a special dietary regimen" and implies that water drinking and cod liver oil were the main items in that regimen, the article states clearly "there was complete curtailment of soft drinks, candy, cake, ice cream or any food made up of white sugar. . . . Those who felt that the sacrifice of coffee was too great were allowed black coffee—fifteen minutes before breakfast."

So we have a group of 98 arthritics starting on a six-month diet in which they are allowed nothing that contains white sugar and, most of them, no coffee. It's not hard for us to believe that such a diet produced almost miraculous improvement in their physical condition, but it is hard to believe that the cod liver oil and the pattern of water drinking were the main reasons for the improvement.

Here are the diet rules which the arthritic patients observed. (1) All daily intake was of water consumed upon arising, preferably at warm temperatures and about one hour before breakfast. (2) Room temperature milk or warm soup (not creamed) were the only liquid permitted with meals. These were allowed any time. (3) Cod liver oil, mixed, either with two tablespoonfuls of fresh, strained orange juice or two tablespoonfuls of cool milk, was taken on a fasting stomach at least four, but preferably five or more, hours after the evening meal and before retiring, or one or more hours before breakfast upon arising and at least one-half hour after water intake. Diabetics and people with heart disease took the oil only twice a week. The cod liver oil mixtures were shaken well in a screw-top glass before taking.

(4) Tablets, pills or supplements of any kind were allowed either with water upon arising, with milk or soup at mealtime, or with milk or soup at any time. (5) No sugar or any food made with sugar. (6) No coffee except before breakfast.

It is our belief that such an experiment is not really a proof of any of the various things involved —the oil, the water, the food supplements which were allowed or the restriction of sugar. It is a test of all these. We would have something worthwhile in the way of scientific research if the two Massachusetts physicians followed this up with a six-month experiment in which the patients eat exactly as they had been eating before, but take cod liver oil as directed and regulate their fluid intake as directed. Then we want to see another six-month experiment in which mixtures of cod liver oil and water drinking are ignored and patients are put on a sugar-free diet *with no other restriction* —and are permitted to take food supplements. Until someone proves us wrong, we are expecting to see improvement on *this* kind of a diet.

It seems to us a harmless enough thing to experiment with different patterns of water drinking. We know perfectly healthy people who never drink water at all, but depend entirely on the ample fluid in their fruits and vegetables to keep themselves from drying out. We know other people – healthy, too – who drink water any time they feel thirsty.

Sugar is highly concentrated, remember, with all the water removed. This is why it cakes so easily in a damp climate and absorbs water thirstily. So of course, anyone who includes in his meals lots of food made with white sugar will want water and will probably want it while he is eating, because the sugar is absorbing water from his tissues which must be replaced. Start him on a sugar-free diet and see his thirst decline!

Here are some other interesting comments from this very provocative article by Drs. Brusch and Johnson in the *National Medical Association Journal.* They state that cholesterol levels dropped or could be controlled, even with the introduction of milk, eggs, butter and cod liver oil. "*For many patients in the study these were new foods,*" they say.

Such a comment shows clearly that these fatty foods (all fats from animal origin) did not cause a rise in cholesterol content of the blood. On the contrary, the cholesterol content of the patients' blood had become high while they were not eating these foods, and was lowered when these foods were given to them on this special diet. We know that fish liver oils, although they are animal rather than vegetable in origin, contain the valuable unsaturated fatty acids which apparently help to emulsify cholesterol so that it does not collect in the blood.

Our thoughts on the Cambridge experiment are: If you want to try the suggested water drinking program and cod liver oil taking, by all means go ahead. It couldn't possibly do you any harm. But please do consider the most important recommendation of Drs. Brusch and Johnson to be their positive prohibition of any foods made with white sugar and their strong recommendation to give up coffee.

Other suggestions for dietary treatment of arthritis are given in a book called *Degeneration-Regeneration* by Melvin Page, D.D.S. (published by Biochemical Research Foundation, 2810 First St., North, St. Petersburg, Fla.). In Dr. Page's view, the whole source of arthritic problems lies in the occurrence of an imbalance in the calcium-phosphorus ratio of the blood. The ideal proportions, says Dr. Page, are a level of 10 for calcium against a level of 4 for phosphorus in a blood test reading. Any alteration of these proportions can lead to trouble.

The body chemistry can be affected by several types of conditions. Mental stress can cause an upset in the chemistry and bring on strong arthritic symptoms via aching joints, that will disappear with the relief of the worry. Certain mechanical conditions can be the cause. If, for the example, normal blood flow is impeded by bad sleeping habits or posture faults, arthritis can result in the affected area. This theory was proven in experiments with animals in which circulation was deliberately impeded in a certain limb, resulting in arthritic conditions in that limb.

The calcium-phosphorus proportion is normally agitated by infection. Dr. Page found that many cases of arthritis could be arrested by eliminating a source of infection. One of the chief sites for infection was found to be the stumps of tonsils which had not been completely removed. The infected part that was left was overgrown with scar tissue, cutting off the chance for drainage. However, Dr. Page cautions against the automatic diagnosis of infection in every case of arthritis. Many good teeth, as well as gall bladders, tonsils and other possible seats of infection have been needlessly removed by doctors who acted on suspicion rather than evidence. Strangely enough, almost every operation leaves the patient greatly relieved of the arthritis symptoms because, says Dr. Page, the healing process following the operation serves to raise the phosphorus level to a balance with the calcium. This relief is short-lived if the operation was not founded on an actual need and the arthritis is soon back again.

Another common cause of upset in the proper balance of calcium and phosphorus in the body is menopause. The glandular changes that take place at this time are often enough to upset the body chemistry to the extent that any incipient arthritic condition is aggravated into showing its symptoms. Though we do not necessarily approve of Dr. Page's treatment, in this instance, we think it only fair to report that he suggest that female sex hormones and insulin be ingested for relief of pain. Also, a tablespoon of molasses or honey after each meal may be used to raise the phosphorus level and ease the pain, in the early stages of arthritis.

Dr. Page says sugar will have the same effect. However, the food values in honey and molasses make them much more desirable in this case.

The best cure for arthritis of all kinds is a diet that will reverse the depleted efficiency of body chemistry, Dr. Page says. He calls it "Biologic Diet."

In his work with arthritis, Dr. Page found that most sufferers from the disease eat similar diets. Usually they consist of high amounts of carbohydrates, low trace mineral intake, and low consumption of foods rich in vitamin B. The large amount of white sugar ingested displaces by its large calorie count, an equal amount of calories from foods that contain the elements the body needs. Sugar is the surest means of knocking the calcium-phosphorus balance out of kilter. It always boosts the calcium count while lowering the phosphorus, then when the effect has worn off, the reverse occurs, with the phosphorus shooting up and calcium becoming depressed. The elimination of sugar, along with white flour and alcohol, both of which have a similar effect, is considered by

Page the most important step in the cure of arthritis. That alone he says, should put the arthritic on the road to cure, but further insurance lies in abandoning completely the use of refined and processed foods. These foods seem to contain many elements which adversely affect the calcium-phosphorus ratio in the blood.

A case cited in the book describes a woman of 52 who became arthritic. She ate a typical American diet, laced with six cups of coffee (1 tsp. sugar in each), plus two cocktails and a highball every day. Besides this she ate candy, cookies and canned fruits—all of which contain white sugar. When tested, her calcium-phosphorus balance was perfect; 10-4. This phenomenon was due to the specious effect of the large amounts of sugar she ate, and as soon as she eliminated sugar from her diet, the calcium-phosphorus level dropped to its true figure—8.4 calcium, 4 phosphorus. After two months on the Biologic Diet the calcium went up and in three months the proper level for calcium and phosphorus had been reached without the artificial prop of sugar, and best of all, the arthritis had disappeared.

Dr. Page warns that response to this treatment may take more time in some individuals than in others. Usually those whose families are relatively new to American diet have faster results than those whose family trees are American from away back and have been steeped in bad dietary habits for generations.

A further contribution to the anti-rheumatism diet is made by Dr. Robert Bingham of California, whom we quoted at the beginning of this chapter. Talking before the 1967 annual seminar of the American Nutrition Society in Pasadena, California, Dr. Bingham expressed fully and convincingly a point of view which he summed up in a quotation from the brilliant, pioneering dentist Weston A. Price:

"Applied nutrition in everyday life is the only way a human being may avoid arthritis and it is the first and best step for a patient to take to treat his arthritis."

Bingham agrees completely with Price. In the first place, it would be difficult to dispute Price's findings which have since been confirmed by dozens of independent studies, that wherever there is a group of isolated people, whether primitive or otherwise, whose diet is abundant in natural unprocessed foods and sufficiently varied to supply all necessary nutrients, there is not a single case of arthritis to be found. This, in itself, is not conclusive proof since the way of life of such isolated and usually primitive people is in many respects besides diet different from that of more civilized and arthritic people. But Dr. Bingham goes on to point out that to any specialist in disorders of bone it is apparent that nutrition plays a major role.

"Diseases of the bones and joints which are due to deficiencies in a single nutritional factor are many. They include scurvy, a vitamin C deficiency; rickets, vitamin D deficiency; osteoporosis, from a lack of calcium and protein; neuropathy, from vitamin B complex deficiency; and degenerative joint disease due to a combination of nutritional deficiencies." He points out furthermore, that these same nutritional deficiencies open the door to many of the infectious diseases by lowering the natural resistance of the body to bacteria, viruses and parasites. This further emphasizes the relationship of nutrition and arthritis, he says, because "Secondary arthritis is often caused by diseases which interfere with the absorption, digestion and metabolism of certain vital nutritional factors." Such diseases include disturbances of the digestive system, food allergies, endocrine (glandular) diseases and the changes in body chemistry associated with the menopause and the aging processes of the body.

Bingham goes on to point out that while gross nutritional deficiencies can be recognized by the medical practitioner, "Subclinical deficiencies, usually too small to be detected by ordinary means, usually multiple in their existence and occurring over a period of years may bring on more subtle changes in the bones and joints and result in degenerative bone and joint disease, commonly called osteoarthritis or hypertrophic osteoarthrosis. This used to be considered a disease of old age, but in our era of 'civilized foods' with its increased use of nutritionally poor foodstuffs we are seeing this condition in more and more young people and are not surprised to find it in the 30's and 40's where our medical authorities taught us to expect it in the 60's and 70's."

Once arthritis has developed, Dr. Bingham does not believe that all patients can be helped by nutritional or any other means, although he does feel that the major portion of the medical profession would be amazed to learn how many arthritics can be helped by nutritional measures. It is in the area of prevention of arthritis, however, that he believes truly good nutrition coupled with a healthful life can be completely successful.

By a reverse process, Dr. Bingham has attempted to isolate the specific factors that enter into resistance to arthritis, and lack of which permit the disease to develop:

"First is under-nutrition. This is usually the result of ignorance, neglect and poverty." And by examination and analysis of children suffering from an early form of rheumatoid arthritis he finds that the deficiencies involved are "deficiencies in vitamin C, the B complex vitamins, calcium, vitamin D and iron. Iron deficiency anemias are found in 10 per cent to 15 per cent of both the younger and older groups. Poor iron absorption from deficiencies in the B complex vitamins, gastric acidity and the trace minerals associated with iron are found. . . . In spite of the fact that generations ago vitamin D deficiency was so well recognized that all children were given cod liver oil, today the propaganda about 'good wholesome food' and dependence on intermittent administration of multiple vitamins has increased the number of cases we have seen with vitamin D deficiencies and rickets. The reliance of some families on prepared milk and processed foods has so decreased their natural vitamin C content that in some areas, particularly in Canada, vitamin C is now added to evaporated milk."

Over-nutrition, Dr. Bingham points out, is also a great problem. "Our sedentary occupations, more riding in automobiles than walking, foods high in sugar, starches and fats have produced an overweight population, particularly in women and older people. The human digestive system, being naturally lazy, absorbs these simple types of foods more quickly and completely than it does the proteins which may or may not be in normal supply. As a result the average elder person is deficient in bone and muscle protein, bone calcium, good joint cartilage and is overweight with excessive fat deposited in the tissue, the body organs and the arteries. Osteoarthritis or degenerative arthritis of the joints is basically a disease of poor circulation to the joints. The increased weight and increased fat associated with arteriosclerosis provides a basis for gradual joint destruction before the patient is aware that much of this has occurred.

"Third, environmental dangers to nutrition, such as pesticides in foods impaired by smog and even radioactive fallout are becoming hazards which must be carefully watched and studied.

"Complications of nutrition caused by toxic medications, the cortisone drugs, medications for ulcer remedies for constipation, pain-relieving and tranquilizing medications and even the antibiotics can adversely affect the patient's digestion or absorption of necessary nutrients from foods."

Thus, Dr. Bingham summarizes his nutritional treatment as bringing the patient to attain a normal body weight, increasing proteins in the diet and reducing carbohydrates and fats, increasing the use of natural and live foods "to introduce the maximum quantity of vitamins, trace minerals and enzymes," and the use of mineral and vitamin supplements and digestive enzymes and food concentrates where necessary.

It is an admirable program that has been found to work out not only by Dr. Bingham but by every doctor we know of whose mind has been sufficiently open to permit him to try it with his patients. There is no point at which we would disagree with Dr. Bingham, although we do wish that he had put more emphasis in his presentation on the role of calcium deficiency in causing arthritis. In September, 1953, Dr. L. W. Cromwell of San Diego, California reported to the Gerontological Society in San Francisco that he found calcium deficiency a major cause of arthritis.

Calcium deficiency, he said, leads first to a condition of osteoporosis (demineralized bones) which is not necessarily apparent, unless the sufferer happens to break a bone. Because of the depletion of bone calcium, the body compensates by depositing extra calcium that causes the stiffness, the pain and the inflammation that are typical of arthritis.

Thus, an important part of everyone's program to keep himself free of arthritis should include regular supplements of bone meal in the diet. Bone, it is apparent, contains not only calcium but also all the other gross and trace minerals such as phosphorus and copper, that aid the absorption of calcium and combine with it to form the hardest and strongest bone. Thus bone meal, alone of all the foods we know, gives us all the mineral elements we require to keep our bones from ever demineralizing. It is our best insurance against ever allowing to start the vicious process of bone resorption.

Combined with a substantial proportion of natural, unprocessed foods in a diet fortified with a more than adequate supply of all the vitamins, it should greatly improve the chances that the presently healthy person will never be afflicted with arthritis.

Before we conclude our discussion of diet and its relationship to rheumatoid arthritis, it ought to be pointed out that the disease itself may be the cause of some deficiencies. Iron, for example, seems to be lacking in some cases of rheumatoid arthritis.

If there's anything an arthritic doesn't need it is weakness, dizziness, headaches, palpitations and a constant feeling of tiredness added to the misery of his aching joints. Unfortunately these added discomforts are symptoms of iron deficiency. Women, especially, tend to suffer from faulty iron absorption when they have arthritis, according to experiments by two Montreal physicians reporting in the *Canadian Medical Association Journal* (September 2, 1967).

The doctors, M. R. Vas, M.D. and N. K. M. Leeuw, M.D., rounded up 21 experimental patients with rheumatoid arthritis, and 25 controls. Then they concocted a drink containing an iron compound in carefully measured amounts, and withheld all medications, except steroids, 12 hours before, and 3 hours after the patient drank the iron solution. Then iron absorption was measured. All the patients stayed in the hospital during the investigation, from eight to ten days.

The experiment showed that all of the 14 female arthritic patients had lower iron supplies in their bloodstream than did the controls. Interestingly, there was no significant difference in iron supply between the seven men with rheumatoid arthritis and the 13 healthy men. The women with rheumatoid arthritis absorbed an average of 26 per cent of the test dose, ranging individually from 9 to 68 per cent; the control women averaged 64 per cent iron absorption, with an individual range of 42 to 96 per cent of the test dose. Again there was no significant difference between the male patients and controls.

It was important to discover if there were any of

the more common causes of iron deficiency operating in these patients, before blaming arthritis. A check for iron intake in food showed no evidence of gross deficiency in any of the patients. Occult or rectal bleeding can result in enough blood loss to cause anemia. However, the researchers were convinced that none of the patients had this problem.

Was it the effect of drugs taken to ease arthritis which caused the iron shortage? "It is possible," said the doctors, "that some of the drugs that the patients were taking interfered with iron absorption either by formation of insoluble complexes. . . or by affecting the intestinal mucosa. There was suggestive evidence that chloroquine decreased iron absorption in one patient. No definite correlation could be established between salicylate intake and iron absorption. . . ." Later the authors reported their observation that iron absorption in an iron-deficient woman with rheumatoid arthritis rose from 32 per cent to 82 per cent after withdrawal of salicylates (aspirin) for 48 hours.

While the exact mechanism is elusive, it is fairly certain that iron absorption is impaired in some persons who have rheumatoid arthritis, and that the impairment is more likely in female patients than in male patients (although some researchers found decreased iron absorption in four of seven male patients under the same conditions).

The importance of iron in maintaining human health is hard to exaggerate. It is a vital component of hemoglobin, the oxygen-carrying compound in the blood. Iron is found in the enzyme system that works to produce energy and it appears in the muscles as a part of the protein that absorbs and reserves oxygen. A large percentage of iron in blood plasma is utilized in the bone marrow to make more hemoglobin and form more enzymes.

On the average, the adult body contains about 4.5 grams of iron. About a gram of this is stored principally in the liver and the spleen. But we all lose some iron every day by way of sweat, hair, cells that break down in the skin and the mucosa, urinary and fecal excretions. The normal iron loss for a man is about a milligram every day; for a women it goes up to 14 to 28 grams a day during menstruation, and 300 to 500 milligrams of iron are lost during pregnancy. A woman's loss during her active sexual life is estimated at one to two milligrams of iron a day. To replace these losses, estimates are that the daily iron intake for adult men and women must be between 10 and 20 milligrams, since only about 10 per cent of what is ingested is absorbed.

If you are arthritic the need for concern about your iron intake and absorption is obvious. If you are taking any of the steroids or chloroquine or aspirin on a regular basis, you have every reason to be especially concerned about how much iron you get in the foods you eat. Make it a special point to include some of the organ meats in your menu several times a week. Liver, heart, and kidney are rated highest in iron content of all the meats. If you are less than fond of them, desiccated liver offers an easy and reliable way around the problem. It contains all of the iron in liver that appears on your plate, without the taste and texture which some people simply cannot abide. Beans, seeds, nuts and other legumes, along with wheat germ and dried fruits, are all good iron sources. Milk is not; and this is why many doctors advise parents to introduce egg yolk, meat, and green leafy vegetables into infant feedings as soon as possible.

Because iron is so vital to so many basic body functions, many healthy people insist on some supplementary source of this mineral every day. Such insurance is particularly important for anyone suffering from arthritis.

Arthritics, and other chronically ill persons who use cortisone over periods of years, are also liable to a B_6 deficiency. In a study involving a large number of hospitalized children being treated for rheumatic fever with massive doses of cortisone, it was observed that they all developed rampant dental decay. Strean says that the stress of the crippling disease plus the large amounts of cortisone interfered with the availability of pyridoxine to the tissues of the children.

It is one more reason why liver or desiccated liver, both excellent sources of the B complex of vitamins, should be regularly included in the diets of all arthritics.

CHAPTER VI

Mineral Baths and Physical Therapy

MINERAL BATHS are still highly recommended by some doctors in treating rheumatoid arthritis—and they are undoubtedly one of the oldest therapies known.

"Heat in almost all forms is highly desirable. The types of heat may vary with each case . . . hot water bottles, heating pads, hot packs or compresses, warm baths . . . give a lot of help." So says the Arthritis and Rheumatism Foundation in a leaflet *What You Should Know About Arthritis.*

Comments Walter S. McClellan, M.D., writing in *The Cyclopedia of Medicine, Surgery, Specialties,* "The treatment of a patient with *rheumatoid arthris* with physical medicine including heat, massage and exercise stands out as one of the most universally valuable forms of therapy. Hydrotherapy (baths) offers a valuable adjunct both for the provision of heat and a medium for exercise."

Since the beginning of history people have used mineral baths to treat diseases. Mineral springs, you know, are springs in which considerable amounts of minerals occur naturally; the springs in Yellowstone Park are examples. And of course there are many natural mineral spring spas in various parts of the country which were popular health resorts not so long ago. You went to the spa to "take the cure" or to "take the waters." You drank or bathed in the water, or both.

The popularity of the spa has declined in this country. The main reason for this seems to be that wealthy people (the only ones who could afford to "take the waters") began to look elsewhere for treatment of their diseases, as well as the elaborately organized social life that went along with "taking the waters." The fancy hotels began to crumble, there was not enough business to pay for repairs and eventually the whole idea of a healthful vacation at a mineral spring became passé.

Besides, during the past fifteen or twenty years, we had the wonder drugs, so the milder and less dramatic methods of treatment ceased to appeal. Who wants to spend a couple of months getting rid of the pain of arthritis, when he can get a shot of cortisone in five minutes?

But the wonder drugs have not been successful in treating the rheumatic diseases. True, some of them can control symptoms for brief periods, but the disease goes right on and may even become much more serious without giving the patient any warning that this is so.

In the case of the rheumatic diseases, then, it seems wise to reconsider one of the old, time-honored methods of treatment which can certainly do no harm and, judging from the material we have read, may accomplish a lot of good. Hot baths relieve many kinds of pain. We all know this. We know that a hot bath can loosen tight muscles and relieve aching joints when we have overworked at some unusual activity. We are told by experts that moist heat is far more effective in relieving pain than dry heat. There are three reasons for this, Dr. McClellan tells us:

1. Increased elimination of waste products through the skin and the kidneys.

2. Improved circulation of the blood and other body fluids, because the heat expands the blood vessels.

3. Mechanical breaking down of adhesions and softening of any thickening in muscles and tissues.

The effectiveness of a hot bath depends on how much of the body is submerged, how hot the water is and how long the patient stays in the bath.

Stiffness of joints is perhaps the most troublesome characteristic of the rheumatic diseases. Anything (such as moist heat) which will loosen these joints and permit freer motion is beneficial. Keeping the muscles inactive tends to cause them to become less and less usable. This leads to less and less activity, more and more pain, and decreased mobility.

Is there any value in taking mineral baths rather than just plain water baths?

We think there is. Apparently the minerals – at least some of them – are absorbed through the skin. In 1929 three researchers at the Mayo clinic published in the *Archives of Dermatology and Syphilology,* volume 20, page 158, their findings on the absorption of sulfur from sulfur baths. They found that all of the subjects had increased sulfur in their blood after the bath – some of them four times as much.

We know that sulfur is important for the efficient working of the human body. It is present in every plant and animal cell. In the body the muscles contain about half the sulfur, while bones and skin contain most of the rest. Foods high in protein are also high in sulfur, for it is contained in several of the amino acids or forms of protein which are absolutely essential to human welfare.

Is it possible that the arthritis patient may be lacking in sulfur? And the sulfur supplied by the bath helps to make up this deficiency? We are told that in a test conducted by two researchers and reported in the *Journal of Bone and Joint Surgery,* (volume XVI, page 185, 1935), it was found that the cystine content of the fingernails of arthritic patients is far lower than that of normal subjects. Cystine is one of the forms of protein which contains a lot of sulfur. It has also been found that the cystine content of the fingernails increases after a sulfur bath.

Are the good effects of mineral baths perhaps just the result of the hot water and the relaxation that goes along with the bath? Apparently not, for researchers have tested patients with and without minerals in the baths and have found that the mineral baths produce better results than plain water, even though they do not know what the reason is.

A series of tests was recently done by several New York physicians. Sixty patients, all of whom were suffering from one form or another of rheumatic complaint, were given a mineral preparation of which the chief ingredient was sulfur and were instructed to use it in a 20-minute hot bath every night just before going to bed. Another 60 patients were instructed to take hot baths consisting of plain tap water.

The results showed that in the 60 cases treated with the sulfur preparations there was relief from pain in 51 cases, no relief in 8 cases, and an increase in pain in 1. Relief of pain was complete in 27 cases. Among those who took the plain hot baths, there was relief of pain in 42 cases, no relief in 17 and aggravation of pain in 1. Relief of pain was complete in 15 cases. In many cases patients who had trouble sleeping found they could drop off to sleep with no trouble, after a sulfur bath.

In no case was there any difference in the amount of movement possible for the affected limbs.

Another interesting experiment was performed at a United States Veterans Hospital at Saratoga Springs where some 1,000 veterans with arthritic symptoms were given mineral baths. Of these 26.3 per cent were slightly improved, 52.2 per cent were moderately improved and 8.7 per cent were markedly improved. Only 7.8 per cent showed no change. A report on this experiment in *Rheumatic Diseases*, prepared under the auspices of the American Rheumatism Association said, "the program built around mineral waters and associated treatments, particularly when occupational therapy and corrective exercise are included can be of real benefit in the rehabilitation of many patients with arthritis. . . . The way in which mineral waters produce these effects must have further study before it can definitely be stated that any specific chemical or agent in the water is responsible for any particular response in pathologic physiology."

Although physical treatment of the many types of arthritis never should be used to the exclusion of other therapeutic procedures, it nonetheless plays a very important part in modern treatment. Most aspects of physical therapy can be applied in the patient's own home, according to Frank H. Krusen, M.D., writing in the *Journal of the American Medical Association.* But Dr. Krusen insists,

"Whereas it is possible to bring great benefit to a patient who has arthritis by the utilization of certain simple physical measures as a part of the home treatment, such procedures can be used to greatest advantage only when they are made a part of a well-planned program of general treatment."

One type of physical therapy is thermal or heat treatment. There are many simple devices for generating heat, among them clamp lamps to be fastened to the back of a chair, the edge of a table or the side of a bed, a homemade "baker" consisting of curved sheet tin with electric sockets attached to the undersurface, hot paraffin packs, natural or artificial sunlight, wet packs and hot tub baths. In some cases it may be more effective to alternately immerse the affected part of the body in cold and hot water.

Massage or manipulation has also been given a great deal of attention in arthritis therapy. It improves circulation, removes excess fluid or swelling from the tissues and can restore flexibility to joints and muscles. Massage may also relieve pain, promote relaxation and leave the patient with a feel-ing of well-being.

These guidelines should be kept in line by anyone giving a massage to an arthritic:

The technique depends, of course, on its purpose and the condition being treated. In general, the movement should be slow, rhythmic, smooth, and toward the heart, Gentle stroking of the skin may help to reduce swelling and improve local circulation.

Tissues which are bruised or are infiltrated with blood must be massaged with particular care. And if there is any possibility that a blood clot has formed, massage ought to be avoided altogether. Otherwise, the clot can be loosened into the bloodstream, plug an artery and cause death.

To help to soothe tight or painful muscles, a deeper stroke with a kneading motion is required. But if the muscles are paralyzed or damaged, they must be massaged gently. In such cases, it is advisable to get medical supervision first.

Never massage if infection is present. Rather than easing pain, you will increase it—not to mention that you may spread the infection to other parts of the body. The same is true of tumor growths.

Dr. Krusen suggests that doctors treating arthritics make it a point to instruct a member of the patient's family in the art of massage. Chances are, the average doctor will not bother to do it, however, unless you ask him.

CHAPTER VII

Exercise and Rheumatoid Arthritis

FOR THE PERSON suffering from painful rheumatoid arthritis, movement of any sort is the last thing in the world he wants. Ironically, there is evidence that movement—lots of it—may be a big help in relieving his suffering.

According to the Arthritis Foundation, "Exercises are extremely important. The Foundation says in its publication, *Rheumatoid Arthritis, A Handbook for Patients,* "It may seem unreasonable in a disease that attacks joints and makes them stiff and sore, but it does make a lot of sense. Rheumatoid arthritis is an illness that tends to make joints stiff, and even to restrict their motion, especially if they are not used.

"It is usually after a period of maintaining the same position that joints in rheumatoid arthritis feel particularly stiff and painful, and this is especially true if it has been a long period. The patient with rheumatoid arthritis tends to be stiff and to feel pain early in the morning, right after arising. It is when he exercises and works the stiffness off that he begins to feel better. A long automobile ride, where the patient sits in one position for an hour or several hours, can also bring on stiffness. It is not true, however, that working out will get rid of arthritis.

"In rheumatoid arthritis, there is the danger that the full movement of individual joints will be lost. For example, if a patient has a knee affected by the disease, he may find that he cannot quite straighten out that knee. This narrowing down of the range of motion can come rather quickly, sometimes before the patient realizes it is happening. Although there are methods for improving the motion of a joint that has become restricted, they are not always effective, and it is much better to prevent reduced motion in the first place.

"What kind of exercise is the doctor likely to prescribe?

"There are a great many, and it is not likely that he will prescribe all of them. Some are called active exercises and are done by the patient without any physical help from anyone, but often under the supervision of the doctor or physical therapist. Others are called passive exercises, in which a doctor or therapist moves the arm, hand, or leg, or whatever part may be involved, but the patient does not exert any effort.

"Assistive exercises are those performed by the patient with the help of a physical therapist or another person trained by a licensed therapist. Exercises of this kind are used to increase the range of motion of a joint and strengthen muscles. The patient, for example, may not be able to fully straighten his arm, but with a little help he may be enabled to do so. The improvement will not come in one exercise session, but perhaps over weeks or even months.

"Sometimes the doctor may prescribe resistance exercises. In these the patient works against some kind of extra force or pressure. An individual may push his foot against pressure applied by the hand of some other person, or he may use exercise apparatus with weights or springs. Exercises of this kind are used particularly to build up strength in weakened muscles.

"Exercises should not be painful, or at most only slightly so. It should be emphasized that exercises are most effective when combined with a complete treatment program.

"If a person continues the usual daily activities are exercises really necessary?

"Yes, one may be told by the doctor that he may continue the usual job or other activities, perhaps even sports and that this general activity will be helpful. But some activities result in sharp and sudden strains on joints and must be avoided. Most daily activities or games do not in themselves give the kind of motion through the entire range of a joint's swing that is so important. The exercises your doctor will prescribe may, for example, include a special kind of clenching and unclenching of the fist, an undramatic and quiet sort of thing that does a great deal of good, and might never occur in one's occupation or in athletics. It would be wonderful if the patient were allowed to do the exercises he enjoys most, but then, how he exercises in daily activities may be quite different from the gentle but effective treatment-exercises the doctor may recommend.

"Does the doctor always prescribe exercise?

"It is not 100 per cent sure that he will. There may be certain periods in arthritis when the doctor may not prescribe exercise. All treatment, whether it is exercise, rest, drugs, surgery—or whatever it is—depends on the particular condition of the patient, and the doctor must make an individualized judgment on what should be done. But exercise is almost always a part of the treatment used at some time or other today."

A final theory is that rheumatoid arthritis may be related to foot disability. As we have already explained, the cause of rheumatoid arthritis is still unknown. It is uncommon though, where people go barefoot or wear non-deforming footgear. In most cases a postural factor can be demonstrated before the onset of this disease. In its later stages it causes permanent damage and contraction of the various joints, making any movement difficult and free use of the hands and feet often impossible.

Women outnumber men in the ratio of three to one in contracting the disease. It may be pointed out that, in considering foot disability as a cause, we find that also more common among women. The typical person contracting rheumatoid arthritis is between the ages of twenty and forty, inclined to be asthenic, chronically fatigue-ridden, with poor posture and imbalance, and strained feet. The usual history then reveals that such an individual is subjected to a physically stressful period when joint coverings become actively inflamed and the disease first manifests. If the strain continues, the disease progresses at a rapid rate. However, in many cases in which the patient has recognized the postural source of the illness and avoided undue stress or use of the feet, the progress of rheumatoid arthritis has become subdued.

CHAPTER VIII

Arthritis—An Emotional Illness?

IT MAY STRIKE you as incredible and far-fetched at first. Nonetheless, there is a growing amount of convincing evidence to support the theory that some cases of arthritis are traceable to friction, discontent and frustration in family, social or business life.

In a paper presented before the General Meeting of the Indiana Medical Association and published in the *Journal* of that society in 1945, Dr. Loring T. Swaim, of Boston, Massachusetts, said that **rheumatoid arthritis** is the direct outgrowth of disturbance to the emotions, manifesting itself in an inflammation in the membranes and tissues surrounding the **smaller joints** (usually those in the fingers, wrists, elbows, ankles and metatarsal arch of the foot). If not arrested, extensive deformities result, their ravages accounting for most of the bed-ridden and wheel-chair confined arthritics. But its greater perniciousness does not consist only in the fact that it twists and warps human bodies more cruelly than does osteoarthritis — it also plays its merciless game with bodies of younger people.

Dr. Swaim's first step in diagnosing and treating this type of patient is to take a complete personal history, or what he calls a "three-way history." The "Laboratory Check" is only one part of his record, for he stresses the fact that emotional disturbances play a significantly large part in the prevention and cure of this disease. Part Two of his patients' records he calls the "Relationship History," one which in his own words "correlates the setbacks in the disease with the emotional reactions to various adverse episodes in the patient's business or family life, such as quarrels, financial reverses, moves to new surroundings, deaths — all the things that make or break us, according to how we take them. Interesting, too, are the habits of eating and sleeping, thinking, and acting that are conditioned by family living. Is the patient's home and business life congenial or strained, happy or tense?"

Part Three of the record is called a "Spiritual History." The most deeply probing of the three, it endeavors to bring to light the beliefs by which the patient lives. "Do his beliefs really affect his thinking and actions, especially towards the people closest to him, or are they purely intellectual? Is his security in material things and self-effort, or has he a sustaining faith which carries him through the emergencies of his life?" Firmly convinced that most people fail to see the connection between their inner spiritual selves and their outward physical persons, Dr. Swaim has come by his convictions from the fact that an astonishingly large proportion of the patients he has treated show a definite connection between their physical ailment and their attitude toward life. If their spirits were secure and satisfied, he found very little joint reaction, but as soon as insecurity and dissatisfaction showed up, they experienced frequent flare-ups of their joints. In fact the very first symptoms of their arthritic condition often occurred immediately after a siege of family trouble. He emphasizes that "the future course of the disease is determined by the kind of character they have developed over the years."

In his course of treatment, he begins with strong doses of rest, since the rheumatoid sufferer is always tired and underweight. The hospital is the best place in which to administer this medicine, inasmuch as these patients, being at least semineurotic to start with, do better away from their familiar and usual surroundings. Posture exercises are also in order, as a tired person invariably falls into poor body positions. Moist heat applications, hot fomentations, and massage are beneficial therapeutic aids.

Dr. Swaim stresses the importance of both the

physical and mental environment of the patient. The home must be heated and sunny, the afflicted person must dress warmly, and his place of work must not be detrimental to his health. Chill, dampness, or exposure either at home or at work must be guarded against, and in climates in which such adverse weather conditions are inevitable, a change of location should be recommended to any rheumatoid sufferer. The food which his family eats is also to be checked in the case of an arthritic: does it consist only of meat, bread, and potatoes? Or are ample fruits and vegetables a regular part of his daily meals? Habits of rest and sleep must be established to provide sufficient doses of relaxation for bodily repair. In general, it is especially important in the case of an arthritic to correct any and all unfavorable conditions as much as possible.

His mental atmosphere may well determine the recovery of this type of patient. In a test study of 50 cases, Dr. Walter Bauer found that 66 per cent of them showed a direct correlation between disturbing episodes in their lives and the flare-ups of their sickness. One-half of the cases confessed to frustration and unhappiness at home. Dr. Swaim found an even bigger percentage of maladjustment and discontent in the case histories of his patients. Reporting that unhappy personal relationships and derivative fear and resentment resulted from the selfishness characteristic of this type of patient, he states that emotional upheavals in the forms of bursts of passion invariably undid all the benefits they had secured by having their condition treated. "Some change," he says, "had to take place in the patient and his home life in order to prevent these setbacks; otherwise, ultimate improvement was uncertain and limited."

That is where the "spiritual history" he takes from each of his patients comes in handy as an indispensable tool. It supplies the foundations on which to erect a new outlook and a healthier approach to life. Sometimes a change-of-heart is in line not only for the sufferer but for his whole family as well. They must learn to cooperate and share mutual interests, to fit into their environment as a constructive force, not a negative and destructive one. Having followed this course of psychic rehabilitation in the case of his patients for the last twelve years, he has had abundant evidence to prove his contention that homes in which there is constant friction should be as much the concern of the medical profession as any other part of its treatment.

Appalled by the number of unhappy homes in America and by the amount of sickness of mind and body they are producing, Dr. Swaim considers it to be the duty of himself and all his colleagues in the medical profession to intervene and mediate in such dissension-torn homes. Such intervention for the sake of mediation he calls "preventive medicine at its best." Concluding that 70 per cent of the patients whom medical science is asked to treat show no organic malfunctions or disease, he finds this high prevalence of psychic upset to be indicative of the world's alarming need for a new spirit. With admirable sincerity and foresight he poses the question whether the next great advance in medicine may not have to come from each and every doctor himself, when as an individual the entire profession shows itself willing to "assume the responsibility of bringing this spirit to a sick world."

Swaim's theories about arthritis and the emotions are not original with him. There are studies on the subject that were conducted as early as 1935.

Just about all researchers agree that arthritis is the result of many physiological factors, but the evidence we've seen is significant enough, we think, to make the inclusion of emotional upsets a part of the list.

An article in the *Canadian Medical Association Journal* (September 15, 1957) says rheumatoid arthritis is a "stress disease and represents a maladaptation to psychobiological stress." Or, more simply, a severe emotional problem can lead you right into a case of swollen joints and arthritic misery.

The authors discuss previous research and study along these lines and summarize the findings of the past 20 years. It is emphasized that these conclusions can only be classed as generalized, due to the many uncontrollable factors involved in dealing with individual emotions and attitudes that have been shaped by a million impressions over a lifetime. It is amazing, though, to see the similarity of personality development in the arthritic individuals studied. Briefly, here are the findings up to now: In 1935, a study showed that arthritics seemed to try to escape from emotional conflicts through physical function. A study involving 32 patients led the observer to note that "a fairly severe emotional disturbance of one kind or another had been present before any sign of rheumatoid arthritis was observed."

A very common emotional mark in rheumatoid arthritics was noted by Halliday in 1937 and 1942: rheumatoid arthritics show a definite restriction of emotional expression as well as strong elements of self-sacrifice. This impression is backed up by a 1954 study which concluded that rheumatoid arthritis seems to follow events which upset the balance between aggressive impulses and their control. For example, let's say a man is unhappy in his job, but knows that he must keep it for the sake of his family's welfare. His resentment against his circumstances might never be spoken outright. But an unjust reprimand might lead to arthritis. This is the kind of circumstance we mean.

It seems to be of major significance in supporting the emotional stress-to-athritis theory to note that there is a relative absence of arthritis among those who are actually adjudged insane. It would seem that these people have given up the struggle to control the repressions and frustrations which are believed to manifest themselves in arthritis.

These brief summaries are contained in the above mentioned Canadian journal as a preface to the detailed description of a similar study. Eighteen arthritis patients were studied. The problem was to get 18 nonarthritics whose background was as similar as possible, to act as controls. The solution lay in using the brother or sister of the patient, as close in age as possible and of the same sex, if that was possible. This procedure also would reduce hereditary differences. The age of the subjects ranged from 20 to 60 years.

All of the people, both arthritics and nonarthritics, used in the study were interviewed by a social worker, to determine their physical environmental background, both in the past and at present. They each spent from 3 to 10 hours with a psychiatrist, who attempted to acquire an accurate picture of their individual personalities and mental attitudes. And finally all were given objective psychological tests.

The general findings of the examinations were these: In childhood the arthritic patients had shown impulsiveness and love of strenuous activity—sports and games, etc. The brothers and sisters of these people showed an opposite tendency in childhood; they were quiet, shy and obedient to the point of envying the boisterousness of their brothers or sisters.

As adults these characteristics reversed themselves in the people observed. The arthritics had restrained their activity in games and sports (not necessarily due to invalidism) as though answering some inner compulsion. They were obsessed with the need to be tidy and punctual, etc. Any aggression they'd shown as children was now replaced with self-sacrifice and forgiving attitudes.

And what of the non-arthritic brothers and sisters? Of course you've guessed it: they became aggressive, full of self-confidence, and free of shyness as adults.

In the interviews an interesting physiological fact was revealed. Many of the arthritis patients had experienced other psychosomatic ailments such as eczema and migraine headaches preceding the onset of the disease.

A classic example of psychosomatic arthritis is Betty Aldrich. She is in her late forties, married and the mother of two children. Like many other married women, she feels that life is nothing but a series of quarrels with her husband, problems with the children, frustrations with bills, meals and household chores.

The way Betty sees it, she has given unselfishly of herself from the first day of her marriage 15 years ago—and in exchange has received nothing but abuse. Her husband is hypercritical, thoughtless and inconsiderate. Many are the nights Betty cries herself to sleep while George watches the late show.

When disagreements develop, Betty does not argue. She keeps her feelings bottled up inside and broods over them for days.

In addition to the problems with her family and with herself, Betty Aldrich also has a physical problem. Recently she began suffering from a severe case of arthritis. It has grown rapidly more severe, and she is now partially crippled by it. Medical therapy has not helped.

Betty's story is a sad one, but it is not unique. For in recent years researchers have begun to recognize that there is a definite relationship between personality and the development of arthritis.

Recently George F. Solomon, M.D., an assistant professor of psychiatry at Stanford University, announced his still far-out theory that arthritis, with all of its physical pain and physical deformities, could actually be related in some way to a "negative" personality.

One of the few men to share Solomon's view at that time was Dr. Sidney Cobb of the Institute for Social Research at the University of Michigan. Cobb studied 97 couples and concluded that wives are more likely to develop rheumatoid arthritis if in their marriages there is continual bickering than if there is a less strenuous relationship.

Except for scattered reports like this, the literature on arthritis and the mind is virtually nonexistent. In May, 1968, the same Dr. Solomon who pioneered in the field made a more detailed report on it. He presented his views at the Second Conference on Psychophysiological Aspects of Cancer before the New York Academy of Sciences.

Solomon is one of a body of researchers who believe that arthritis is an auto-immune disease. That is, it is related to the body's own immunity system. When foreign bodies such as bacteria or viruses enter the body, the system sends out antigens to meet the invaders. When the antigens clash with the foreign bodies, they produce antibodies, the actual substances which surround and destroy the invaders. In arthritis, it is possible that antibodies are never produced against the invading viruses, so those viruses lodge in the joints to cause trouble. Another theory is that the antibodies are produced, but are unable to differentiate between the enemy viruses and the healthy cells. As a result, they destroy both. According to this theory, the body's own defense system causes arthritis.

Solomon believes the first theory is the true one. He suggests that certain emotional patterns may affect hormonal balance, and that this in turn may lower a person's ability to produce antibodies against viruses or whatever else the cause of arthritis may be.

To support his theory, Solomon referred to the work of a fellow researcher. He told the New York Academy of Sciences in May, 1968:

"Moos' review of the literature of over 5,000 patients with rheumatoid arthritis found that investigators agreed that arthritics, when compared with various control groups, tend to be self-sacrificing, masochistic, conforming, self-conscious, shy, inhibited, perfectionistic. . . ."

Following the issuance of the Moos report, Solomon teamed up with Moos to conduct a further investigation. He chose a group of women and gave them the Minnesota Multiphasic Personality Inventory, a test designed to probe the basic personality make-up of people.

The results were persuasive. Unlike most others, the women with arthritis who took the test were invariably nervous, tense, worried, moody, depressed, concerned with what they considered rejection from their mothers and strictness from their fathers. Instead of having occasional outbursts of anger such as most people experience, the arthritic women inhibited any expression of emotion. They showed tendencies to comply and to be subservient. They had great need for security, were shy and introverted.

Solomon then carried out another study including "rheumatoid factor" as an element to test the relationship between arthritis and personality.

A good deal of interest has been generated of late concerning the role "rheumatoid factor," a substance found in the blood of rheumatoid arthritics, plays in the development of the disease. Solomon, too, was interested in answering that question. He said, "We compared two groups of healthy female relatives of rheumatoid arthritic patients, one group having, and the other lacking rheumatoid factor in their sera (blood). . ."

His study showed that, if it is true that the rheumatoid factor plays a part in the development of arthritis, it is equally true that the state of emotional health is also important. The healthy relatives who had the rheumatoid factor were most frequently well adjusted and with positive outlooks on life. Those healthy women who suffered from anxiety, depression, low self-esteem, alienation, fear and worry were—fortunately—lacking in the rheumatoid factor. This perhaps explains why they were not suffering from arthritis.

Solomon concludes, "It seemed as if the occurrence of psychic disequilibrium (emotional upset) in the presence of rheumatoid factor might lead to overt rheumatoid disease. . ." If a person is physically healthy, he says, but possesses the rheumatoid factor, he must make sure he maintains psychological health as well if he is to avoid arthritis.

While carrying on the study, Solomon made another discovery—accidentally. He found that certain women seemed to improve with medical care, while others grew progressively worse and ended up crippled just as Betty Aldrich did. This, too, according to Dr. Solomon, was at least partly the result of personality. Solomon says a progressive worsening of an arthritic condition is caused by "unsuccessful ego adaption." What he means is this:

When people are faced with emotional or psychological changes, they react to them in many different ways. For example, when embarrassed, one person may routinely react by laughing. Another may become angry. Another may simply shrug. The way we adapt to various situations in order to save face is called "ego adaption." Each of us has a whole set of ego adaptions. The healthy person chooses positive adaptions, but the arthritic, according to Solomon, reacts negatively. When embarrassed, the arthritic will probably keep his feelings bottled up inside and will brood over the embarrassment for days or weeks.

With some people, the method of ego adaptation resorted to is not sufficient to do what it is meant to do. It does not save face. It does not restore a feeling of self-sufficiency or personal worthwhileness.

Solomon's study suggested that the people with inadequate methods of ego adaptation are the ones who grow progressively worse with arthritis, eventually ending up crippled.

Is arthritis caused by a rheumatoid factor? Is it caused by the body's own antibodies attacking healthy cells? Is it caused by viruses the body is not capable of warding off? Nobody can yet answer those questions. But one point that can be made with some assurance is that arthritis is directly related to a defeatist outlook. The person who sees nothing but the storm clouds and never glimpses the silver lining is the potential arthritic.

Another study on the same subject is outlined in the August 15, 1967 issue of the same periodical, *The Canadian Medical Association Journal.* The author in this case states at the outset that emotional or psychological factors are usually listed among the causes of rheumatoid arthritis in standard textbooks dealing with this disease. Also it is said to be common that flare-ups and relapses of the disease often follow emotional stress from various sources.

Studies of 43 chronic rheumatoid arthritis patients yielded some interesting generalizations. For example, a majority of the patients associated the onset of the disease with the death of a spouse, separation from a spouse, prolonged separation from a family or leaving home to become established—all situations which carried in them the elements which could be woven into great emotional stress. Add to this the traits of immaturity, dependence, concealed hostility and excessively insistent cooperation in everything, and you have a picture of the average arthritic in this study.

This information does not imply that any person to whom such unfortunate things happen will end as a rheumatoid arthritic. Most persons who lose parents, who end an unhappy marriage in divorce or separation or who meet with frustration in beginning a career do not find themselves victims of this disease. Somehow or other they must have accumulated inner resources to battle against such a breakdown. Even though the trigger of stress was pulled, it did not bring about a physiological breakdown. No one can be sure he is possessed of such resources but we can all do our best to see that our bodies have the raw material to manufacture the nutritional blocks against arthritis.

CHAPTER IX

Gout

WHAT IS A gout attack like? The doctors who have seen one call it: "Torture!", "Agonizing!", "Unbearable!", "Excruciating!" To the victim words like these seem pale and inadequate. After all, they attempt to describe several hours, sometimes several days, of white hot pain that begins so suddenly and is so intense that it often shocks the victim right out of a deep sleep.

If the misery is in the bunion joint (it usually is —though any joint is vulnerable) it will be swollen in no time and have an angry, shiny reddish-purple appearance. Very, very tender. Bed clothes lying on it will feel like a ton of needles; the most painstaking change of position is enough to bring tears. The patient will hardly notice the chills and fever and heart palpitations that always go with acute attacks of gout.

When the acute phase of the attack has passed, the pain goes and the patient may have 6 months, and perhaps several years, without an attack. But one attack means a second attack is almost a certainty. A few really unfortunate gout victims seem to acquire the habit, and acute attacks become more and more frequent over the years.

One of the classic descriptions of a gout attack in medical literature is Sydenham's 17th century masterpiece.

"The victim goes to bed and sleeps in good health. About two o'clock in the morning he is awakened by a severe pain in the great toe; more rarely in the heel, ankle or instep. This pain is like that of a dislocation, and yet the parts feel as if cold water were poured over them. Then follow chills and shivers, and a little fever. The pain, which was at first moderate, becomes more intense. With its intensity, the chills and shivers increase. After a time this comes to its height, accommodating itself to the bones and ligaments of the tarsus and metatarsus. Now it is a violent stretching and tearing of the ligaments—now it is a gnawing pain and now a pressure and tightening. So exquisite and lively meanwhile the feeling of the part affected, that it cannot bear the weight of bedclothes nor the jar of a person walking in the room."

Benjamin Franklin also wrote of gout. In November, 1780, Franklin had a very bad siege of the gout that lasted about six weeks. During that time he wrote his celebrated "Dialogue Between Franklin and the Gout." Here it is:

"Let us examine your course of life," the Gout said. "When the mornings are long and you have plenty of time to go out for a walk, what do you do? Instead of getting up an appetite for breakfast by salutary exercise you amuse yourself with books, pamphlets, and newspapers most of which are not worth the trouble. Yet you eat an abundant breakfast, not less than four cups of tea with cream, and one or two slices of buttered toast covered with strips of smoked beef.

"Immediately afterwards you sit down to write at your desk or talk with people who come to see you on business. This lasts till an hour after noon, without any kind of bodily exercise.

"But what do you do after dinner? Instead of walking in the beautiful gardens of the friends with whom you have dined, like a man of sense, you settle down to the chessboard and there you stay for two or three hours.

"Wrapped in the speculations of this wretched game, you destroy your constitution.

"Do not flatter yourself that when you ride for half an hour in your carriage you are taking exercise. Providence has not given carriages to everybody, but it has given everybody a pair of legs.

"Remember how often you have promised yourself to walk tomorrow morning in the Bois de Boulogne, in the garden at La Muette or in your own, and then have not kept your word; alleging sometimes that it was too cold, at other times too warm, too damp, or too something else; when in truth it was too much nothing which hindered you but too much laziness.

"You know M. B.(rillon)'s gardens and how good they are for walking; you know the fine flight of a hundred and fifty steps which lead from the terrace down to the lawn. You have been in the habit of visiting this amiable family twice a week in the afternoon. A maxim you yourself invented says that a man may have as much exercise in going a mile up and down stairs as in walking ten on level ground. What an opportunity for you to take exercise in both these ways!

"What have you done? You have sat on the terrace, praised the fine view, and looked at the beauties of the gardens below; but you have never stirred a step to descend and walk about in them. On the contrary, you call for tea and the chessboard.

"And then, instead of walking home, which would stir you up a little, you take your carriage.

"*Franklin*: What would you have me do with my carriage?

"*Gout*: Burn it if you like.

"Or, if that proposal does not suit you, I have another. Observe the poor peasants who till the soil in the vineyards and fields about the villages of Passy, Auteuil, Chaillot, etc. Every day you may find among these good creatures four or five old women and old men, bent and perhaps crippled by the weight of years and by labour too hard and unrelieved, who after a long, fatiguing day have to walk a mile or two to their cottages. Order your coachman to pick them up and take them home. That will be a good deed, and good for your soul! And if at the same time, after your visit to the B(rillon)'s, you return on foot, that will be good for your body.

"*Franklin*: Ah! how tiresome you are.

"Oh! oh! for heaven's sake leave me! and I promise faithfully that from now on I shall play no more chess but shall take daily exercises and live temperately.

"*Gout*: I know you too well. You promise beautifully; but, after a few months of good health, you will go back to your old habits; your fine promises will be forgotten like the forms of last year's clouds."

Ben Franklin is one example of a widely-held theory that gout and greatness go together. For centuries, sufferers with the gout have consoled themselves with Sir Thomas Sydenham's judgment: "Gout attacks more wise men than fools." This theory has persisted even to the present. Recently it turned up as a basis for a project of the Survey Research Center at the University of Michigan.

Students have been impressed by the fact that the disease is commonly mentioned by biographers and frequently encountered among people of distinction and achievement, says the University of

Michigan report which appeared in the *JAMA* (February 7, 1966). The possibility that uric acid, the source of gout problems, might serve as a stimulant to the cerebral cortex was proposed by E. Orowan in *Nature* (April, 1955). It was his idea that the superior intelligence of man and primates is due to the comparatively high levels of uric acid in these animals.

George W. Brooks, MPH, and Ernst Mueller, Ph.D., found in social class evaluations some evidence that "Perhaps a tendency to gout was a tendency to the executive suite." To make their own determination of this Brooks and Mueller interviewed 122 men in academic positions. The results were rather interesting: "We believe. . . that such possible stimulation (high uric acid levels) has a much stronger relationship to achievement orientation in our culture than it has to high scores on intelligence tests." In other words, the high uric acid level is related more to drive than intelligence.

The history books are loaded with evidence for equating gout with achievement. Many heroes of Greek mythology were said to suffer from gout—King Priam of Troy, Achilles, and Oedipus, King of Thebes. Some great figures of the Italian Renaissance were gout victims. The entire Medici family is a good example. According to *A Short History of the Gout* by W. S. C. Copeman, "Lorenzo the Magnificent, who although he inherited the family gout, was less severely afflicted than his father and grandfather and lived to enhance the Medician patronage of the arts, of which Michelangelo, another sufferer, was the chief glory." The Holy Roman Emperor, Charles V, was almost continuously physically incapacitated by gout for the last eight years of his life.

Sir Francis Bacon, the Lord Chancellor of England, suffered with gout along with his doctor, the great William Harvey, who discovered the circulation of the blood. Historians of the time tell us, "Harvey was much and often troubled with the gout and his way of cure was thus: He would sit with his legs bare, if it were frost, on the roof of Cockaine House, put them in a pail of water till he was almost dead with cold then betake himself to the heat of his stove; and so 'twas gone."

Among the literary figures who suffered with the disease were Dr. Samuel Johnson and the great poet Milton. Milton was tormented by the gout in addition to his blindness and it has been suggested that inspiration for his vivid description of the torments of hell in *Paradise Lost* might have been derived from his disease.

With such well known figures to reinforce the association between accomplishment and the gout, psychiatrist Havelock Ellis wrote, "It is impossible to regard it as not having a real association. . . genius is not a product of gout, but it may be that the gouty poison acts as a real stimulus to intellectual ability and a real aid to intellectual achievement."

Ellis' words are interesting, and may even offer

some half-hearted consolation to the gout sufferers. But they do not, of course, alleviate the pain—not to mention the longer-range problems. For doctors know that many of the 300,000 to 500,000 Americans plagued by gout face serious crippling of the joints all over the body, along with kidney complications that can be fatal.

In fact, the authorities say that kidney disease is quite common in chronic gout. When we discuss what causes gout, we will understand why the kidneys are affected.

Gout victims also have an increased incidence of high blood pressure, and they suffer from it at an earlier age. There are also suggested associations between gout and arteriosclerosis and diabetes mellitus. Major causes of death in gouty patients are heart attack, kidney disease and stroke.

According to the Arthritis Foundation, gout results because the chemistry of the body is out of kilter, resulting in more uric acid in the tissues than there ought to be. In an acute attack of gout, crystals of monosodium urate, a salt of uric acid, form in certain joints. These sharp-edged crystals cause the inflammation and severe pain associated with the disease.

Sometimes these crystals also form in the kidneys and cause perhaps fatal kidney disease.

Normally there is nothing wrong with uric acid. It is found as a waste product in every human being. It is produced from substances known as purines.

Purines are solute crystalline compounds found in many foods, but in especially large quantities in those which are the organs of animals, such as sweetbreads, brains, kidney and liver. Beer is another purine source. All purines do not come directly from the food supply, however; a large percentage actually is manufactured in the body.

When purine-containing foods are digested, uric acid is produced. Normally the body is equipped to destroy or eliminate it. The uric acid is excreted partly by way of the kidney and partly by way of the intestinal tract. What is not filtered out by the kidney is absorbed into the bloodstream to be destroyed by the body's defenders, leucocytes and erythrocytes. In gout victims this mechanism for taking care of uric acid is out of order.

Researchers studying the cause of gout are confronted with two possibilities: the body could be manufacturing an excess of purines, or the body's destructive processes for uric acid could be at fault. No one familiar with the problem is willing to say for sure which it is.

There is an obvious parallel between the purines and cholesterol. Both are contained in the foods we eat and both are also produced by the body. If the body is equipped to synthesize them, presumably there is a basic need for them in the human physiology. This is known to be true of cholesterol, which among its other duties, is needed to nourish the brain.

The body is geared to handle any excess of cholesterol, just as it can take care of excessive uric acid, the by-product of purine. If either mechanism for doing these jobs breaks down, the accumulated excess in the bloodstream causes serious difficulties—circulatory in the case of cholesterol, renal (kidney) and skeletal with uric acid. Researchers have found that the body uses unsaturated fats to thin out its cholesterol accumulations, so diets high in this element plus a cut in cholesterol-rich foods are generally recommended by doctors to combat too-high cholesterol readings. There is still no information on how to stimulate the body's natural ability to destroy uric acid, so the doctors attempt to reduce the amount by recommending a cut in purine-rich foods.

It is puzzling to discover that some of the foods richest in vital nutrients are also high in the purines, therefore bad for gout sufferers. As we have already said, meats, especially the glandular or organ meats are high in purine. So are cereals, dried beans, asparagus, cauliflower, mushrooms, onions, and peas. But so are the fatty meats, pastries, nuts, ice cream and other rich foods. Alcohol, coffee and tea all contain purine.

The most recent evidence against alcohol appears in the *Medical Journal of Australia* (June 17, 1967) in which 157 subjects were tested, 13 of whom had critical gout. The tests showed what the investigation termed "highly significant correlations with alcohol consumption, particularly of beer." Highly significant also were the correlations of gout with tobacco consumption. A causal relationship between regular alcohol consumption and gout is suggested, and the desirability of avoidance of all forms of alcohol by gout subjects is reemphasized.

Of course the purine pile-up presents no problem to the non-gouty individual. Organ meats, nuts, and fresh or dried beans are loaded with nutrients we all need. One simply cannot afford to eliminate these items from the diet on the off-chance that gout lies somewhere in the future. Foods such as fatty meats, pastries, and ice cream create many difficulties that have nothing to do with their purine content, so health-conscious people with or without gout avoid them altogether.

Do you have to wait for that day of misery to know that you are gout-prone? Not at all. Your doctor may include a uric acid analysis of your blood in your regular check-up. (In men over 35 and women over 50, this is especially important, since these are the beginning ages of gout.) The reading should be no more than 6.3 milligrams per 100 milliliters; if it is higher, the tendency toward gout must be suspected. The records say that about 2 per cent of the population as a whole has above-average uric acid readings. However, in gouty families (it runs in families) it might range up to 72 per cent.

If a patient shows arthritic symptoms, the doctor

should check the uric acid level to be sure it is arthritis and not gout, since the symptoms are sometimes confusing. High uric acid is enough to call for a restricted purine diet, but great care must be exercised to see that the nutrients lost from the meat and vegetables are replaced by non-purine foods and food supplements. You may be able to get along without purine in your diet, but you need the B-complex you lose without organ meats, and the vitamins A and C that are lost with the vegetables you eliminate.

When gout has progressed for a while, lumps and bumps—painful ones—called *tophi* begin to appear around the joints. They are crystallized uric acid deposits, and they can become so massive as to cripple the joint entirely. They might appear years before any characteristic attack, hence are often mis-diagnosed as arthritis. X-ray can be used to tell the difference.

One of the most dependable therapeutic tools in gout is the use of colchicine, an ancient drug in Cleopatra's time, and still the drug of choice. No one can explain how, but a dose of colchicine will usually relieve an acute gout attack within a few hours. The bulb of the autumn crocus harbors this spectacular herb medication which works wonders on gout—and nothing else.

Gout patients are advised by doctors to go nowhere, and do nothing without a dose of colchicine close at hand. It is to be taken at the first hint of an attack. Definite and quick changes in mood or complete depression that lasts for days, severe fatigue and radical change in eating habits—all are danger signs.

Like other powerful drugs, colchicine requires careful attention to control of dosage. The side effects can be catastrophic in themselves. Patients are warned to discontinue the drug at the *very first sign* of diarrhea, whether the pain has gone or not. Too much colchicine causes nausea, vomiting, cramps, severe diarrhea, vascular and kidney damage, severe dehydration and low blood pressure. As little as 7 milligrams has caused death. And once the poisoning begins, there is no known antidote.

In spite of these hazards doctors frequently put gout patients on daily 2 milligram maintenance doses of colchicine between attacks. The risks of potent drugs must sometimes be accepted in the treatment of serious ailments, and if a reasonable amount of colchicine can bring relief from the agony of a gout attack, its use is certainly justified. But we cannot agree with the AMA's Council on Drugs on using it daily over a period of years, just in case.

Attempts have been made to create drugs that will handle gout by lowering the uric acid content of the blood. Such drugs must be taken on a long term basis and because of this, side effects become increasingly important. The current favorite, Benemid, calls for one or two tablets taken every day to double the amount of uric acid excreted by the body. But, according to the AMA's own evaluation, Benemid ". . . may produce an acute attack of gouty arthritis when used as a urate eliminant in chronic gout. Also . . . it is possible that probenecid (Benemid) may favor the formation of uric acid stones from urates that would tend to crystallize in an acid urine." Since the declared purpose of taking Benemid is to prevent a gout attack and deposits of uric acid crystals, one can't help feeling that Benemid falls short of the ideal. Aside from known gastrointestinal complications, Benemid's full range of side effects has yet to be determined.

Flexin, another drug introduced into the gout group, came a cropper in 1961, when it was withdrawn from the market because deaths from liver damage were related to its use. Actually, Flexin had no curative effect on gout, but worked more as an antipain device. Its use appears to be typical of the groping nature of most modern anti-gout treatments. Only this one happened to have fatal consequences for some.

Another approach to handling gout which has no side effects, and is apparently as effective as at least some of the drugs is described by Ludwig W. Blau, M.D. in an article titled "Cherry Diet Control for Gout and Arthritis" (*Texas Reports on Biology and Medicine,* volume 8, Fall, 1950). Dr. Blau proposed a large cherry intake as effective in the treatment of the disease. Though he adds that "apologies are offered for unsatisfactory clinical and laboratory data and control," he feels nonetheless that the discovery merits the "propriety of publishing the information available."

Twelve cases of gout responded so favorably to this food that the blood uric acid of the sufferers dropped to its usual average and "no attacks of gouty arthritis have occurred on a non-restricted diet in all 12 cases, as a result of eating about one-half pound of fresh or canned cherries per day." Supporting his evidence with details concerning three of these cases, Dr. Blau demonstrates the relief brought by the eating of either canned cherries, sour, black or Royal Anne, or fresh Black Bing varieties. In one case the juice only was drunk, and this proved to be about equally effective.

At first it may seem incredible that so ordinary a thing as cherries could prevent attacks of one of the most painful ailments known. Yet, here is what one former gout sufferer, Col. Ike Ashburn of Austin, Texas, has to say:

"At Mayo's (Clinic in Rochester, Minn., where he went because of intolerable suffering from gout), the gout man told me when I asked him whether there was any merit in the eating of cherries to prevent recurrence of gout, that if I found that it worked for me, I should by all means continue eating them.

"It has been just about a year since I had any recurrence, though I had a number of pretty severe attacks for at least a couple of years before. I am careful not to bruise the foot, but I have had no excruciating pain for nearly a year.

"I eat just about every day some of the common old pie cherries. . . . I have at least half a dozen friends who have just about warded off their gout attacks by reliance on cherries."

D. T. Hicks is another who can dramatically attest to the effect cherries had on his gout.

"I entered Scott and White Hospital in Temple (Texas) in a wheelchair last January," he writes, "suffering the tortures of the damned. And I walked out a week later free of pain. I had not connected the cherry juice that they gave me with gout treatment. . . ."

Eight years later, in *Food Field Reporter* for November 10, 1958, appeared an article on canned cherry juice relieving arthritis. Says the *Reporter,* new evidence that canned cherry juice may relieve gout, gouty arthritis and similar ailments is reported by Reynolds Brothers, Inc. at Sturgeon Bay, Wisconsin. According to the article, a number of residents of Sturgeon Bay cooperated in testing the cherry juice daily. "Outstanding results were reported," said the president of the firm who sold the cherry juice. He says further that sales of his product have increased considerably in Texas since the article appeared there linking cherry juice to arthritic cure. He also disclosed that several local dentists have been suggesting cherry juice to their patients and one of them found it useful for the treatment of pyorrhea.

"To date," says *Food Field Reporter,* "there is no definite scientific data on just how the juice aids in relieving pain caused by diseases where improper balance of calcium is evident. However, it is believed that it may be the pigment in the cherries that brings relief."

In Morris B. Jacobs' standard reference work on foods, *Food and Food Products,* we read that cherries contain several pigments. They also contain quite a concentration of malic acid and a surprising amount of pectin. That is the substance in fruits that is used to make jelly harden and "jell." There are also small amounts of citric acid, oxalic acid, succinic and lactic acid in cherries. The oxalic acid exists in only trace amounts, fortunately, for this is a substance very destructive of one's calcium supply. Surprisingly enough, there is also a small amount of linoleic acid in cherries. That is the unsaturated fatty acid which apparently has such a powerful effect on the body's use of the fatty substance cholesterol.

In this information there seems to be no clue as to what element of the cherry may be effective against gouty arthritis. It would certainly be a challenging experiment for scientists to work on. And we are sure that any of the thousands of gout sufferers would be more than willing to act as guinea pigs for such an experiment, if there was the slightest chance that he might be relieved of his symptoms.

Meanwhile, what can readers who are suffering from gouty arthritis do about this information? Canned cherries are of course available in grocery stores everywhere. Most brands are loaded with sugar, probably also artificial coloring matter and other chemicals. The cherries themselves were of course sprayed with insecticide and on a small fruit like this which is not peeled, these insecticides can mount up to a frightening total.

If you have cherry trees or know anyone who does, by all means freeze or can some next Spring for your own use. If you get very sour cherries you can use honey for the processing. Remember that honey has almost twice the sweetening power of sugar, so judge the amount you use accordingly.

Among the strangest therapies ever offered for gout was one by Dr. Thomas Sydenham, the father of English medicine, whose description of gout we quoted earlier. Sydenham believed in many natural ways to cure diseases—especially *horseback riding*. He found it effective in phthisis, gout, and abdominal pains. Dr. Paris, who wrote about Sydenham, said of this treatment: "This great physician, Sydenham, having long attended a gentleman of fortune, with little or no advantage, frankly avowed his inability to render him any further service, adding, at the same time, that there was a physician of the name of Robertson at

Inverness who had distinguished himself by the performance of many remarkable cures of the same complaint as that under which his patient labored, and expressing a conviction that, if he applied to him, he would come back cured. This was too encouraging a proposal to be neglected; the gentleman received from Sydenham a statement of his case, with the necessary letter of introduction, and proceeded without delay to the place in question. On arriving at Inverness and anxiously enquiring for the residence of Dr. Robertson, he found to his utter dismay and disappointment that there was no physician by that name nor ever had been in the memory of any person there. The gentleman returned vowing eternal hostility to the peace of Sydenham, and on his arrival at home, vehemently expressed his indignation at having been sent on a journey of so many hundred miles for no purpose. "Well," replied Sydenham, "are you better in health?" "Yes, I am now quite well; but no thanks to you." "No," says Sydenham, "but you may thank Dr. Robertson for curing you. I wished to send you on a journey with some object of interest in view. I knew Robertson and his wonderful cures in contemplation; and in returning you were equally engaged in thinking of scolding me."

If we try to look for a reason why the horseback ride cured the man's gout, we might find something. After a few moments of exercise, when the body warms up, it begins to make cortisone. This is natural cortisone, not the synthetic kind that is given for arthritis, of which gout is one form. The young person who is continually on the go has a continuous supply of cortisone. When he gets older and stops exercising, the body gets little of it, and things begin to happen.

Although it may not be feasible for most gout sufferers to go horseback riding, the same effect can be obtained through an exercise program strenuous enough to encourage the body to produce its own cortisone. Such exercises as walking, tennis, golf, and square dancing are good.

In the last analysis, gout occurs because the body isn't working as it should. And this is the clue to its prevention. We have only one tried and true method for maintaining general good health, and that is to nourish our bodies properly. A program which calls for a high protein, low carbohydrate, low fat intake, with no processed foods, is certainly best for that. It considers what the normal body needs to stay healthy and supplies the need. This includes a metabolism that can handle uric acid without creating any problem. No uric acid problem, no gout.

If gout should threaten you, or if you've already had an attack, you'll need this kind of program more than ever.

If overweight, the patient should be instructed in a diet designed gradually to achieve and maintain optimal body weight. A high fluid intake is essential and should be encouraged to minimize the risk of formation of calculi. Alcoholic beverages, coffee, and tea are permitted. Some patients are able to identify foods or beverages which almost invariably precipitate acute attacks. These, of course, should be avoided.

Because you must cut out high purine foods, you will need a guide to a good diet that will supply the precious nutrients you've lost. Consider natural food supplements as your most effective insurance. Eat plenty of eggs. They are low in purines, but still offer plenty of protein. And concentrate on safe fresh vegetables to fill in the vitamin gaps left by those you've had to eliminate. We'll choose this kind of preventive action over daily doses of dangerous drugs every time.

CHAPTER X

Osteoporosis

One of the commonest symptoms of aging, and one of the most difficult for those who suffer it, is increasing brittleness and fragility of the bones. No general hospital is ever without its cases of elderly people who have fractured arms or legs as the result of a fall, and are confined to hospital beds for months waiting for the exaggeratedly slow healing process to take place.

This weakness of the bones of the elderly is due to a condition known as osteoporosis, a loss of weight and density in the bone cells and the development of a spongy rather than a solid texture. It is the leading arthritic disease in the aging.

The disease actually consists of an *enlargement of the spaces in bones* so that its appearance becomes porous. What looked before like a rock now appears like a sponge, with holes growing larger all the time. Since bones are important chiefly for support, you can easily see what difficulties would result. A backbone that cannot support the weight of its owner will produce pain, undoubtedly. Bones which are full of air holes are more likely to break in a fall than solid, staunch bones. Hence the many incidents of broken hips, arms and legs among older people whose steps may be unsteady or whose sight may be dim.

When osteoporosis strikes, the victim will in most cases be a woman, probably over 50. She may have no advance knowledge that she is suffering from the disease, with bones that have been growing more porous and weaker every day for years. Perhaps she will be cleaning the house. She will bend over to dust a table, and a quick, natural movement of her head will cause a bone in her neck to fracture. She may be shopping. Merely stepping from the street to the curb could be enough to splinter the bones of her ankle.

Osteoporosis is one of the most common plagues of advancing age. About one of every three women and one of every five men over 50 who seek medical care have the disease, which is basically a structural weakness of the bones. In later years metabolic factors can interfere with the normal bone re-building process, so that old tissue is lost and no new tissue is formed. The bones grow thinner and weaker.

Backache is the commonest symptom of osteoporosis. The pain will be constant, and will increase when the patient gets up or moves about. Coughing, sneezing and pushing may also increase the pain. Pain may also occur in the joints of the body as calcium, not used in building solid bone, gathers in the joints instead. Victims tend to keep their backs rigorously fixed and walk carefully. Symptoms such as these should be a sign, especially to those over 50, that osteoporosis may have developed.

Until recently osteoporosis was seldom detectable by x-ray till an estimated 30 to 50 per cent of the calcium in the skeleton was lost. By that time the damage was almost beyond repair.

Now doctors detect the disease early by measuring the way sound travels through a bone in the forearm. An acoustical technique determines the density of the ulna bone. The less the density, the more advanced the osteoporosis. This detection method is three to five times more sensitive than x-ray.

An article by B. E. C. Nordin, M.D., which appeared in *The Medical Press* for February 10, 1960, speaks of the causes of osteoporosis. He says that the condition affects far more women than men, possibly because of the greater proportion of older women in the population. Although this ailment may occur at any age it is especially common in older age groups. Supposedly there is relationship between the occurrence of osteoporosis and the menopause. However, we do not know very clearly just what this may be. One reason for its much greater incidence in women appears to be the demands made by childbirth. In one survey which was done, it was found that in a certain group of patients 40 per cent of those women who had not borne children had osteoporosis against 72 per cent of those who had borne many.

Another possible cause of osteoporosis is the drug cortisone. Through experiments with 44 asthmatic patients (*American Journal of Clinical Nutrition,* March, 1965) two Swedish physicians demonstrated that a remarkable number of osteoporosis cases develop in those patients treated with cortisone. The incidence of osteoporosis among asthmatic patients is generally high, perhaps because cortisone is so often used in treating them.

It is also known that one reason the bones fail to rebuild is that formation of the needed protein is no longer stimulated by lagging male and female hormones. This is a paradox—at least on the surface: administering hormones of certain types can also produce osteoporosis.

A drug that can control conception for one year was tested on 350 women at birth control clinics in Mexico City and at the University in Santiago, Chile. A hormone is injected into a muscle and stored there, slowly seeping into the bloodstream which carries it to the body's master gland, the pituitary. It acts on the pituitary to shut down completely the release of hormones that trigger the ovaries to produce hormones.

A woman deprived of these hormones not only becomes infertile but scientists have also found that **osteoporosis** occurs, **along with breakdowns** in elastic fibers of the skin. "This method would be unthinkable in the United States, but in countries where infants must face life-or-death population problems, chances must be taken. . . . The price that must be paid to prevent this will be a million women with soft bones," said Dr. Joseph W. Goldzieher.

In experiments to learn how long the effects of a single shot last, some women receive an injection every three months, some every six months, and some once a year. Goldzieher believes that although the injected hormone causes serious side-effects, the seriousness of the population problem in some parts of the world justifies this method of combating it.

We wonder how many of the women who are participating in these tests fully understand the physical risk they are taking. It is hard to believe that any woman ignorant or not, would voluntarily use a birth control method that is likely to cripple her. Medical ethics that would permit experiments involving such serious consequences are, at best, questionable.

Most researchers are in agreement that nutritional deficiencies play a major role in osteoporosis. Sometimes the relationship is simple and direct. Drs. Jacob Bassan, Boy Frame and Harold Frost in *Annals of Internal Medicine* (March, 1963) state, "Dietary studies in England and the United States indicate that patients with osteoporosis ingest less calcium in their diets as compared with their nonosteoporotic contemporaries." It is obvious. A shortage of calcium means the process of building bone tissue must be impaired. People advanced in age tend to ignore some of the high calcium foods, increasing, instead, their consumption of coffee, cakes and cold cereals, all lacking in nutritive value. They need mineral supplements.

"Patients with osteoporosis eat less calcium and need more than normal people," says Dr. B. E. C. Nordin of Scotland. In *Advances in Metabolic Disorders* (edited by Rachmiel Levine and Rolf Luft, Academic Press, N.Y., 1964) he explains that it is likely the reduced bone mass of the disease is caused by insufficient calcium intake, and inability of the individual to absorb enough of the calcium he is ingesting.

The same point is made in *Arthritis and Rheumatism* (April, 1966, Vol. IX, No. 2, part 1): "In general, the view was favored that osteoporosis resulted from a relative nutritional imbalance of calcium, leading to increased bone resorption. Some osteoporotic patients were found to have consumed diets too low in calcium balance by increasing calcium intake."

The relationship of osteoporosis and calcium, or lack of it, in the diet is clearly shown by the results of many surveys. *The Lancet* for May 7, 1955, reports that in a group of 33 patients over the age of 68 those with a calcium intake under 500 milligrams of calcium daily had a 74 per cent incidence of osteoporosis whereas those who took over 500 milligrams of calcium daily had an incidence of only 14 per cent.

About 99 per cent of the body's calcium is stored in bone. An article by J. M. Finlay in the *Canadian Medical Association Journal* for May 15, 1956, tells us that bone is not a hard, impermeable substance. Instead, all the substances in it are constantly being exchanged, replaced and absorbed into other tissues. The bones of the average person weigh most at about 25 to 30 years of age. Thereafter they decline in weight indicating that minerals are being lost from them.

Whether or not one has enough calcium depends upon three things, according to Dr. Nordin: How much calcium is in one's food, how much one absorbs and how much one excretes. He goes on to say that the average intake of calcium, in England, where he is writing, is 1,000 milligrams of calcium a day. However, he admits that such a figure contains much variation. It is true, he says, that some people do not get this much calcium and still they remain healthy. These folks can apparently adapt to a smaller amount of calcium and not excrete so much in their urine. However, it seems that one's body does not preserve calcium as it does some other minerals. The excretion of sodium can be reduced to almost nothing if one is eating a low-sodium diet. The amount of potassium excreted depends to some extent on how much is taken in. But it appears that the body is quite wasteful of calcium even when you are getting not nearly enough in your food.

"It is possible," says Dr. Nordin, "that the conservation of calcium, of which there are large stores in the skeleton, has been less vital to the organism in evolution than that of sodium, potassium, phosphate and nitrogen." It seems to us that this reluctance of the body to store and save calcium more carefully is an excellent reason to make certain you are getting plenty of it every day.

What about people who don't absorb the calcium they do get? About 15 per cent of these cases suffer from a disorder called steatorrhea, which involves quite distressing diarrhea. In diarrhea, of course, minerals are lost, rather than being absorbed, because they do not stay in the digestive tract long enough to be absorbed.

"The majority of patients with osteoporosis (those with steatorrhea excepted) do go into strongly positive calcium balance when given calcium supplements," says Dr. Nordin. In other words, as soon as they begin to get more than enough calcium, all their calcium needs are taken care of, even though they continue to excrete the same amount of calcium.

However, he goes on, it seems that no matter how much calcium is given, new bone matter is not formed in older people. Taking calcium supplements appears to relieve pain and to stop the progress of the disease, but cannot make any change in the way the bone looks under an x-ray. This may be the reason there is so much osteoporosis these days.

People who, generally speaking, get enough calcium in their food, probably vary their intake from week to week, says Dr. Nordin. When their intake falls below their requirement, their bones suffer, for calcium apparently is withdrawn from the bones. At other times, when they get more calcium, isn't it possible for this part of the bone to be rebuilt? It seems not, says Dr. Nordin, when the people involved are elderly. It is not at all certain, he says, that people beyond middle age have the power to reconstitute this lost bone. So it becomes vitally important for such people to keep their calcium intake high at all times, for harm done by even a short period of having too little can apparently result in damage that can't be repaired.

We think it is startling to find in the pages of a medical magazine a suggestion that even a short period of living on a diet too low in calcium can result in irreparable harm. Surely here is a challenge for real preventive medicine!

Yet, doctors and medical schools generally persist in regarding the development of osteoporosis as one of the many unsolved mysteries connected with the aging process. "Why should the cause of the commonest disorder of the human skeleton, so-called senile or post-menopausal osteoporosis, remain such an enigma?" asks J. Gershon-Cohen, M.D., D. Sc., of the Albert Einstein Medical Center, in an article written by him and several associates in *Radiology* (February, 1962, pages 251-252). To Dr. Gershon-Cohen and his co-researchers there is no mystery about it. Osteoporosis is a loss of calcium from the bones. It would seem obvious that this would be associated with insufficient calcium in the diet. *Lancet,* the English medical journal, has already published studies by Nordin, and Harrison, Fraser, and Mullan, demonstrating that osteoporosis is accompanied by an insufficiency of calcium in the bloodstream. To confirm these findings which the medical profession seems not yet to have accepted, the Gershon-Cohen group conducted a long-term series of experiments on rats. "We found that osteoporosis could be produced in the animals on calcium-deficient diets, within six weeks." This scientific confirmation has been repeated in a number of articles by the same group, published during 1962 in various medical journals.

"More striking was the finding that these osteoporotic animals could be cured of this condition with supplements of calcium-phosphate salts, provided a positive balance was maintained long enough. Normal reconstruction of bones could thus be effected. Roentgenographic (X-ray) chemical and microradiographic studies confirmed these conclusions."

Of course the learned doctors of Albert Einstein Medical Center were seeking experimental evidence of the effect on this degenerative disease of calcium (with its obligatory partner phosphorus). It was necessary for them to use the purified calcium phosphate to avoid the complication of having to account for the possible effect of many other trace minerals. But what they have demonstrated for the pharmaceutical, calcium phosphate, would obviously hold even truer for the natural product bone meal, in which calcium and phosphorus in the same 2 to 1 proportion, are accompanied by the full spectrum of trace minerals that interact with them and make their work more positive and more effective.

Incidentally, that same theory may shed some light on arthritis. In September, 1953, Dr. L. W. Cromwell of San Diego, California, reported to the Gerontological Society in San Francisco that he had found calcium deficiency to be a cause of arthritic crippling. This may seem strange at first glance, since arthritis consists primarily of deposits of extra calcium in the joints of the bones, stiffening them and making movement painful. However, Dr. Cromwell's theory is quite simple to follow and understand.

The calcium deficiency, he says, leads first to a condition of osteoporosis which is not necessarily apparent, unless the sufferer happens to break a bone. Because of the depletion of bone calcium, the body compensates by depositing extra calcium, thus furnishing extra structural rigidity at the points of greatest stress—the joints. Regular consumption of additional calcium, particularly in its most assimilable form—bone meal—by correcting the osteoporotic condition removes the stimulus for the system to keep adding more and more calcium to the bone joints. This gives the body a chance to break down and remove some of the excessive calcium in the joints, thus holding out hope of an improvement in the arthritic condition.

We do not say bone meal will cure arthritis. We do say that if you start young enough and take bone meal supplements consistently, the chances are few and far between that you will ever contract arthritis. And we also point out to the medical profession that treatment of osteoporosis with calcium is a far more sensible approach to the problem of arthritis than the habit-forming, nerve-jangling and useless **corticosteroids.**

We have shown how bone meal serves a valuable preventive function for two of the commonest afflictions that are commonly interpreted as the inevitable result of old age. Osteoporosis and arthritis alone affect at least 15 million Americans. But the relationship of calcium deficiency to "growing old" does not stop there.

In January, 1945, Dr. Ernest H. Planck published in the *Journal of the Medical Association of Alabama* a dissertation on blood calcium and calcium therapy. After a long study, he had found all the following symptoms related to a low level of serum calcium and insufficient calcium in the diet:

1. Bone pain above or below the joints.
2. Cramps in the calf muscles of the leg occurring during sleep or during exercise.

3. Pain in the arms, either in forearm muscles or in the biceps.
4. Painful cramping of the feet and toes after going to bed.
5. Spastic contractions of the hands and fingers after use.
6. Backaches.
7. Insomnia.
8. Dizziness.
9. Nervous irritability and emotional instability.
10. Fainting and nausea in women.
11. Brittle teeth with many cavities.
12. Dermatitis of the scalp and face.
13. Tremors of the fingers.
14. Shortness of breath.

All of these symptoms, which, when they occur in a person past 40 years of age, are commonly considered to be "growing old," and ills for which nothing can be done, were found by Dr. Planck to respond quickly and easily to increased intake of calcium. We ask why anybody should choose to put up with such disorders, when bone meal tablets are so easy and pleasant to take?

Why, then, do all these troubles tend to show up as people grow older? It is not because of increasing age itself, but because as one grows older, the system experiences more difficulty in absorbing and retaining calcium. In addition, one's eating habits tend to change. Older people tend to eat more bread, which contains phytic acid—an antagonist of calcium that carries it right out of the system. Older people drink less milk, which in spite of the many things wrong with it, is a good source of calcium to those who use it. In addition, some have theorized that as people grow older, their stomachs contain less hydrochloric acid, with the result that they have greater difficulty in digesting calcium and more of it is carried out of the system. Too many elderly people try to economize on food, with the result that they cut down on their supply of vitamins A, C and D, all of which, like phosphorus are absolutely necessary, if calcium is to be properly absorbed and utilized by the system.

In other words, a great many ailments, minor or serious, painful or merely annoying, that are generally considered a result of advancing age, are actually a result of advancing age, and are actually a result of depleted stores of calcium in the body. To hold them off or prevent them completely, is as simple as simply increasing the calcium intake every single day, along with the other nutrients that make use of the calcium possible and easy. And it is bone meal that represents the most complete and easiest-to-utilize form of calcium we know.

Some people get plenty of calcium, and still the bones will not harden. Tests show that much of the calcium they get is lost to the body in urine. This may be due to vitamin D deficiency or a need for magnesium. These nutrients help to fuse the calcium into the bones. Doctors sometimes use fish liver oils rich in vitamins A and D in treating osteoporosis, or prescribe diets that include plenty of D-rich eggs, fish and liver.

Two other aspects of osteoporosis are stressed by Dr. Nordin. First the importance of vitamin D for the proper absorption of calcium. Vitamin D occurs most plentifully in fish liver oils, which is why we recommend that they be a part of everyone's daily food supplements. But, in the case of people who cannot absorb vitamin D (diarrhea or other conditions resulting in malabsorption) sunlight is the best source of vitamin D. We do not advise long hours of baking in the sun. The resulting tan means that your body can absorb no more vitamin D. We recommend rather outdoor exercise in the shade, for plenty of vitamin D is around outdoors in the summer. In winter, getting enough vitamin D is a real problem for northerners. Go south if you can. If not, spend as much time as possible outdoors on sunny days. In any case, take fish liver oil, summer and winter, to give the maximum amount of vitamin D.

One other suggestion. Steatorrhea, mentioned by Dr. Nordin as a possible contributing cause of osteoporosis, is frequently involved with difficulties in eating wheat and rye gluten. In other words, it may be the wheat or rye products in one's diet that cause the diarrhea which results in loss of calcium and other precious minerals. If you have any tendencies this way we advise eliminating cereal products from your diet—all breads and breakfast cereals included. Most of us eat far too much cereal anyway, in comparison to the amount of fresh fruits and vegetables, eggs and meat that we eat. If you are suffering from steatorrhea, your doctor has undoubtedly already given you a diet containing no wheat or rye. If not, why not try doing without cereal products for a time just to see if you don't feel better?

Every article that we read on osteoporosis stressed strongly the necessity of physical activity in the prevention and treatment of osteoporosis. Says Benjamin B. Wells in *The American Practitioner and Digest of Treatment* for April, 1956, "diminishing physical activity and loss of muscle strength are undoubtedly contributing factors in senile osteoporosis. Partial or total immobilization of any kind must be combated with every means at our disposal." He also says that studies have indicated that older people need more calcium than younger people to maintain their "calcium balance."

But—to return to this matter of vitamin D—the previously cited *Rheumatism and Arthritis* stresses the importance of that nutrient. In some groups studied, calcium alone did no good. In that study, doses of vitamin D of 5,000 to 10,000 units daily led to a positive calcium balance. Similarly a 23-year-old woman with typical osteoporosis was studied. "This patient was in negative calcium balance (calcium deficiency) on high as well as low calcium intake, but had normal urinary calcium excretion and no evidence for intestinal malabsorption. Positive calcium balance was achieved with large oral doses of vitamin D."

The study continued, "Three female patients (ages 63, 67, and 77) with osteoporosis underwent balance studies for extended periods while on low and high calcium intakes. The addition of calcium gluconate tablets to the low calcium diet improved the calcium balance but not to the extent observed in young persons or in elderly subjects without osteoporosis. *The suggestion was therefore made that patients with osteoporosis have a decreased ability to absorb calcium from the intestine.*"

Another nutrient receiving increasing attention in relation to osteoporosis is vitamin C. An article in the *American Journal of Clinical Nutrition* for November-December, 1957, indicates that chronic lack of vitamin C may be related to this disease. Say the authors, Dr. H. Grusin and E. Samuel, "There is a wealth of experimental evidence to support the view that vitamin C is essential for the formation of osteoid (bone) tissue." This is rather surprising for we generally think of bone only in terms of minerals and vitamin D. And we generally think of bone as being something formed in childhood which does not change from then on. This of course is not the case, for bone reacts to body conditions just as any other part of the body does.

The sixteen patients described in this article were all African Bantus. Perhaps the most revealing aspect of the study is that nine of these patients were suffering from acute scurvy when they entered the hospital. Scurvy is the disease of vitamin C deficiency. Two other patients had either scurvy. So 69 per cent of the patients were or had been scorbutic.

The surprising thing about this fact is that both scurvy and osteoporosis are uncommon diseases at the hospital, yet they were frequently found together in the same patient. The main symptom of all patients was backache. X-rays of spines showed that much calcium had been lost and fractured vertebrae in all cases.

Treatment with vitamin C did not bring the spines back to normal, with one exception. This patient was kept in the hospital for a year and was given a full hospital diet along with rest and massive doses of vitamin C. The other patients continued to eat their usual diet and returned home to hard physical labor (especially carrying heavy loads on their backs) much sooner than that.

The authors conclude that in such an African community there are many factors which might be responsible for osteoporosis. The diet contains little calcium and not too much in the way of animal protein. However, everyone in the community eats this same deficient diet and osteoporosis, as well as scurvy, are found very infrequently. When they do occur, they often occur in the same patient. Say Dr. Grusin and Samuel, "It is suggested that these osteoporotic patients may have suffered from chronic scurvy or minor attacks of scurvy without being incapacitated and that their chronic vitamin-C deficient state eventually led to osteoporosis."

It was those words "chronic or minor attacks of scurvy . . . without being incapacitated" that caught our attention. We have found evidence that many people in America, especially older people, are suffering from these same conditions — minor attacks, or chronic scurvy, evidenced by loose teeth, bruise marks, swollen or inflamed or bleeding gums. In addition, lack of calcium is tragically obvious among our senior population. Could the osteoporosis not be related to these two important deficiencies?

As the doctors in Africa found out, it was not possible to cure the osteoporosis with even large doses (500 milligrams) of vitamin C. But a patient given a good all-round diet and rest, along with the vitamin C, showed improvement. We have in this article only a theory without the painstaking work that is necessary to establish a new principle in nutrition.

But it is enough, we think, to serve as a warning to those of us who are not getting enough vitamin C. Osteoporosis is a painful and often crippling disease. If you can prevent it by eating lots of fruit and vegetables, raw rather than cooked, and by taking additional vitamin C in natural food supplements, don't you think it's worth the effort?

Dr. Wells, whom we mentioned before, stresses

vitamin C. "There is no doubt," he says, "that vitamin C is necessary for the normal mineralization of bone and teeth." Out-and-out scurvy, resulting from complete lack of vitamin C, is rare in old people, but deficiency in vitamin C which we know is very common, must be closely associated with the incidence of osteoporosis, according to Dr. Wells. He also makes one very provocative statement about the possible relation of lessened blood supply secondary to arteriosclerosis (hardening of the arteries) as a factor limiting the production of bone in aging persons. "No positive evidence is available." We'd add—taking vitamin E supplements will lessen the possibility of poor circulation. We would say that vitamin C is extremely important for the prevention of osteoporosis and vitamin C is known to be lacking in most American diets, especially those of older folks—the very ones who need it most. Your richest supply is in fresh raw fruits and vegetables, and rose hips—the concentrated natural supplement made from the fruit of rose bushes.

Consistent protein deficiency can also lead to osteoporosis. According to *Borden's Review of Nutrition Research* (October-December, 1962), "The malnutrition occasionally associated with osteoporosis and occasionally negative nitrogen balance seen in this disorder imply that high protein intake may be of help in treatment." Some researchers suggest that the change in hormone production that accompanies the postmenopausal period affects the protein in some way so that it is not available to the bones.

Finally, Daniel S. Bernstein, M.D. warns in *Postgraduate Medicine* (October, 1963) that a lack of exercise can be harmful to bones. "Osteoporosis of disuse" is well-known in medical circles. It creeps up on older people who don't exercise enough.

Thousands of pages on osteoporosis fill the files of medical literature, yet little more is known about the problem than we have said here. Diets high in calcium, phosphates, protein and vitamin D, combined with plenty of exercise, appear to be the safest and most promising hope for prevention and cure. Supplement the good foods with bone meal and fish liver oils.

Don't wait till the illness becomes obvious. According to some studies, osteoporosis can begin unnoticed at age 30. Encouraged by poor diet, it whittles away little by little. When it is too late to do much about it, there is the unreasonable fracture, the pain and the invalidism.

A new fad gaining some support in certain circles is that fluoride can help in osteoporosis. The evidence—or lack of it—was discussed in the January, 1967, issue of *Prevention*. In an article entitled "Pseudoscience from Harvard," *Prevention* said,

"One of the most blatant attempts to make something out of nothing—specifically to persuade the medical profession on no evidence at all that **fluoridated water will prevent osteoporosis**—was published in the *AMA Journal* for October 31, 1966. The report came out of the Department of Nutrition of the Harvard School of Public Health and is signed by five eminent doctors, any one of whom ought certainly to know the difference between scientific evidence and wild guesswork. One of the five, in fact, is Dr. Fredrick J. Stare who has made quite a reputation as a hard-boiled critic of research by his frequent insistence that evidence be absolutely airtight before *he* will accept it to mean anything at all.

"Yet when it comes to the wild and unscientific schemes to force everyone in our country to drink fluoridated water, suddenly that tough scientific skepticism is thrown to the winds and Dr. Stare seems as willing as any novice to draw conclusions with no substantiation."

Let us examine this so-called scientific report.

The report, in the first place, is based on a study of approximately 1,000 people living in North Dakota. Now this, in itself, is strange. If you wanted to find out the effect of water fluoridation on the development of osteoporosis, it seems to us that you would go to one or more of the pairs of cities that were set up for experimental comparisons of the effects of fluoridation. You might for instance go to Newburgh and Kingston, New York, and see if, after more than twenty years of water fluoridation, there is any less osteoporosis in Newburgh than there is in Kingston.

Such a study would give you well over 100,000

people between whom to make a comparison and to draw statistical conclusions.

Why go to an area so sparsely populated that a bare 1,000 people can be found for a study, and attempt to draw statistical evidence from so few people?

One reason might be that fewer individuals there are in a statistical sample, the bigger are the percentages involved in small and possibly accidental changes. For example, if you have a population of 10,000 people and 100 of them have osteoporosis, the rate is 1 per cent. If you have only 100 people and 5 have osteoporosis, the rate is 5 per cent. In another population of 100, if there are 2 more or 2 less with osteoporosis—something that could happen for entirely accidental reasons—that is a variation of a full 2 per cent.

So we can see that if you were looking for an area where you could gather statistics that would do exactly what you wanted them to do, you might do very well in one offering only 1,000 people to study, and only 339 of them over age 65, which is when osteoporosis becomes a significant medical problem.

In fact, in the high fluoride area of North Dakota that was contrasted with a similar low fluoride area, there were only 80 people of both sexes over the age 65 studied. Really. . . . If you wanted truly to establish whether fluoride in the water would prevent the development of osteoporosis, wouldn't you think you would need more than 80 people over the age of 65 as subjects? For these eminent scientists from Harvard University, however, the 80 were quite enough to serve their purpose.

Commenting to us on the statistical quality of the study, F. B. Exner, M.D., F.A.C.R., a radiologist of prominent standing, said:

"In the first place, they should know and it is clear in the article that they do know that causation can never be inferred from statistics. In the second place, not one of the conditions studied can be determined for statistical purposes by x-ray. In the third place, the films they compared were not even comparable since they were taken by different technicians with different equipment.

"Next, there were far more subjects from the low than high fluoride areas (which, itself, introduces statistical error), plus the fact that the numbers of subjects were too small to mean anything. 32 females aged 55-64, were compared with 120 'low-fluoride' females of the same age; and not all the 32 lived in their counties all their lives. We are not told how long the others had lived elsewhere, or their fluorine-exposure while away. In other words, the 32 is a padded figure, and so were all the others.

"Next, most of the subjects were farmers who presumably used the water on their respective farms. Well-depths in the listed counties are known to range from 7 feet to 1,180 feet. Despite this, the fluorine content of one town in each county is offered as representing the entire county.

"Next, although data are given on how much milk and cheese the subjects consumed, no attempt was made to determine how much water they drank.

"All this would be bad enough if the 'high-fluoride area' had, in fact, been high, and the 'low-fluoride area' low. They were not, and the authors *should* have known it if they did not when the areas were chosen. We are told that levels in the 'high-fluoride area' ranged from 4 to 5.8 ppm. These were the levels in the five highest wells in the counties. Other wells contained from zero to 0.8 ppm.

"We are told that the range in the 'low-fluoride area' was from 0.15 to 0.3 ppm., and the towns of New Rockford, Carrington, and Grafton are listed as representing the three counties. No source for the figures is given; but the authors' 'reference 18' contains a map showing that all three counties are in areas where artesian wells contain 3 to 4 ppm.; and well within the life-times of the subjects of this study.

"Meanwhile, there were veritable 'low-fluoride areas' readily available in North Dakota and where the water-histories of suitable subjects could have been determined. Fargo, Bismarck, Grand Forks, Jamestown, and Valley City, with a combined population of 130,000, all have water supplies with about 0.1 ppm. of fluorine.

"And if the authors had been interested in knowing what *fluoridation,* as contrasted with 'a high-fluoride area' will do, they could have examined subjects in Kingston and Newburgh, New York, where a 'fluoridation experiment' started 20 years ago—although it is still far too early to detect effects which may take 40 years to become manifest."

Now we do not doubt for a moment that the study is a truthful one as far as it goes. That is, we are sure that the figures reported are actually derived from reports by two radiologists, as stated, diagnosing the condition of the vertebrae of all the subjects (though Dr. Exner points out the error in this), and also the amount of calcification of the aorta, the principal artery carrying blood from the heart. What the study found that can be stated as hard fact was that among approximately 1,000 people, 300 living in an area where the water may have had a natural fluoride content of 4 to 5.8 parts per million had lower percentage of osteoporosis and aorta calcification than did 715 living in an area where the fluoride level in the water in some cases was .15 to .3 parts per million.

In such a circumstance, if you had a big enough sample—which you do not—you might then say that you had raised the question of whether *something* or some combination of things in the water *might* bear a relationship to osteoporosis and aortic calcification. In such a case, if you were a scientist, you would then proceed to analyze both water supplies and find out their total mineral content and how they vary, one from the other.

This apparently did not even occur to the Harvard five.

A highly reputable Texas orthopedic surgeon has published studies based on his own long experience in and around Deaf Smith County in Texas. This surgeon, Dr. Lewis B. Barnett, has also found that those who drink water with natural fluoride in it—not artificially fluoridated water—have less osteoporosis. Dr. Barnett, however, made careful analyses of soil and water and read widely in the medical literature, coming to the conclusion that the only mineral from such waters truly important in building resistance to osteoporosis is magnesium phosphate. In Dr. Barnett's opinion, if fluoride plays any role at all in strengthening bone, it is a minor one. Magnesium is the important mineral.

In view of the work of Dr. Barnett, it would be only natural for any doctor reading the report in the *AMA Journal* to ask whether the North Dakota water under consideration contains any substantial amounts of magnesium and phosphorus, and whether there is a difference in the supply of these minerals in the two water sources. No one inquiring about this will find any information in the Harvard study, however. Even though it is well known that natural fluorides occur only in hard water, which is to say water with a varied and extensive mineral content, Dr. Stare's team from Harvard made absolutely no effort so far as can be determined from their report to find out what minerals other than fluoride were in the North Dakota water and whether these minerals might have an influence on bone density. "The purpose of this study," they state, "was to determine whether prolonged ingestion of small amounts of fluoride have an effect on bone density and the rate of progression of osteoporosis." They conclude that it does.

The conclusion is obviously unscientific and unwarranted. But the Director of Medical Information of Harvard University leaped to make capital of it in a nationwide news release sent out even before the article was published. It began by stating: "The prevalence of osteoporosis, a disease in which there is a reduction in bone mass and a fragility of the bones, is lowered significantly in individuals who drink water containing generous concentrations of fluoride.

"This conclusion is drawn by investigators from Harvard's Department of Nutrition. . ."

When scientists conduct a highly unscientific study and reach conclusions whose only value is for propaganda, there is probably a reason and it may have nothing to do with the advancement of medical science. We cannot say what the reason is. It is quite possible that it has nothing to do with the endowments from food manufacturing companies who don't want people to stop eating their sugary foods for the sake of their teeth. We have no way of saying why five eminent men from Harvard University should try to influence the medical profession and the general public by publishing a study which, in our opinion, is a blot on the name of science and the reputation of Harvard University.

The editor of *Rheumatism and Arthritis* comments on the fluoride theory: "The place for fluoride therapy in osteoporosis is still to be established. Although osteosclerosis may result from long-term fluoride ingestion, whether or not this change is beneficial to the patient is not certain. The changes observed in the balance studies reported are suggestive, although not impressive. The proper time to produce increased density of the osteoporotic skeleton with fluoride therapy might be of considerable importance."

"Yet, in the January 28,1967, issue of the *Lancet*, there was an article on fluoride and osteoporosis which jumped on the bandwagon of the Harvard study. This is an example of how medical misconceptions are perpetrated. The *Lancet* said:

"The Harvard inquiry confirms a suspected link between osteoporosis and quite small differences in fluoride intake. A concentration of 4-8 ppm. is, however, too high for use in public water supplies and would result in undesirable enamel defects (mottling) of developing teeth. For dental health in temperate climates such as Britain, a concentration of approximately 1 ppm. is regarded as best, since this confers substantial protection against dental caries, and the incidence of enamel defects is lower than with concentrations both above and below this level.

"In a study of the prevalence of rheumatic diseases in an area where water had been fluoridated at 1 ppm. for five years, Ansell and Lawrence noted less osteoporosis than in a low fluoride control area. The difference, however, was apparent only in women, and Ansell and Lawrence hesitated to attribute the effects to fluoridation. Five years of fluoridation is obviously too little for firm conclusions, but further studies may show more striking differences."

The trouble with this theory is that in this article, the less amount of osteoporosis was observed in areas where the drinking water contained the *natural fluoride.* But in treating drinking water with fluorides the very soluble sodium fluoride is used.

If there was no difference between these *two kinds of fluorides* then people would be killed by drinking river waters with high calcium fluoride content. If there was no difference, people would be killed by drinking tea, or taking bone meal, both of which are extremely high in fluoride content, but it is the non-dangerous calcium fluoride which is almost inert.

We come across this error over and over again.

It is made by doctors, dentists and scientists who never distinguish between these two forms of fluoride.

In summary—vitamin D and C have been proven effective in treating some cases of osteoporosis. Beyond that, protein is very important, and hormones play a part in some round-about way. Yet, hormones used in birth control apparently lead to osteoporosis, rather than treat it. There is no substantial evidence to indicate that sodium fluoride helps.

But the form of therapy which has proven most effective for osteoporotics is a dietary increase of calcium.

Bone meal is your best source of calcium. It is made of powdered bones of young cattle. It contains not only calcium but all the other minerals in bone—phosphorus, potassium, iodine, magnesium and so forth. Take bone meal every day. You can take it in tablet form or, much less expensively, as a powder which you can use in food, in omelets, in fruit drinks, on salads, and other foods.

CHAPTER XI

Fluorosis

DO THESE SYMPTOMS sound familiar: Pain and cramping in the legs or arms or both, weakness and stiffness, excessive thirst, unusual bony growths, frequent fevers, backache?

If they do, it may save your life to know that they are symptoms not of arthritis, but of an arthritic-like disease called fluorosis. Lately, some doctors are coming to realize that more people suffer from it than had been suspected in the past, although it has been known for years that fluorosis is not a rare cause of ailment and death in animals. The *New York Times* reported on January 1, 1968, that the Hooker Chemical Corporation, near Buffalo, Iowa, which produces di-calcium phosphate and a defluorinated phosphate rock for cattle feed supplements, gives off into the atmosphere fluoride-containing dust.

According to three Iowa farmers, Ed Swanson, Ted Porstmann and Omer Seys, that dust has been killing off their livestock. As a result, they have been forced to sell the cattle that remained, and try to raise crops. Yet, the crops, too, have been severely affected by the fluoride dust. Ed Swanson had to dispose of 102 head of livestock, including 48 milk cows. He reported a 25-acre plot that yielded about 2,500 bushels of corn before the plant began operating was reduced to 200 bushels of corn in 1966.

Porstmann farms 140 acres. In 1963 he had a yield of 4,001 bushels of corn from a 40-acre field. That same field raised only 1,600 bushels in 1966. In 1967 it raised only 680 bushels of soybeans. He has had to sell his 12 milk cows.

Swanson said, "We started farming 18 years ago and have been building and working hard all of our lives. We kept adding to our herd and in 1964, I went out of the hog business to concentrate on dairying. It's pretty hard to see your life's work destroyed." Mrs. Swanson is unable to keep plants alive in the house and the family is afraid to eat vegetables from the garden. "We have seen what this stuff does to plants and animals and we worry about what it's doing to our sons," she commented.

Ironically, the Swansons sold the 64 acres on which the plant is situated to the chemical firm in 1963 and the plant began operations in the spring of 1964. The company signed a statement, requested by the county board of supervisors, saying there would be no hazard to the surrounding community as a result of the plant operations.

While the three nearest farms are most seriously damaged, plant pathologists indicate that fluorine damage has been observed on forage as far as 6 1/2 miles east of the plant as well as on farms west and north of the plant, which is bordered on the south by the Mississippi River.

Dr. Orsen Cannon, plant pathologist at Utah State, and Dr. D. C. McCune, plant pathologist for Boyce, Thompson Institute for Plant Research, Inc., in Yonkers, New York, presented the effects on plants and crops after a 3-month investigation of damage, to a meeting of state officials, farmers, and company representatives.

Samples of vegetation and livestock feed tested were found to have a fluoride content ranging from 89 to 1,740 parts per million (30 ppm. is considered "acceptable" for dairy cows).

The fluoride-sprewing feed plant has been recently closed down after the company was presented evidence of the damage. Meanwhile, Dr. William Buck of the Iowa State University's Veterinary Diagnostic Laboratory states that the ultimate effect on surrounding areas of the fluoride—still being deposited on plants—can't be determined until amounts on vegetation are measured this spring.

With mounting reports of damage from fluoride-polluted air, New York State Assemblyman

Chester R. Hardt, in a recent letter to the *New York Times,* gave public voice to his concern over fluoride in the air, and also raised the question of a possible relationship between fluoride air pollution and fluoridated drinking water. Said Hardt:

"I agree that this is the opportune time to take stock of the damage man is doing to his natural environment through pollution of many types.

"In this connection, the writer has vainly attempted to get a reply to this simple question, from the New York State Health Department, Division of Air Resources:

" 'Can it be that our State Health Department takes the position that fluoride contamination of the air is unimportant or that fluoridated drinking water supplies do not contribute to fluoride contamination of the air?'

"When the people of the state and of the nation are spending billions to abate the impact of air pollution—when we have some 90,000,000 chronically ill, and the underlying reasons therefore not known or understood—and with the finger of suspicion pointed at fluoride, an admitted contaminant—I say that immediate remedial action is called for.

"Fluorides enter the body through inhalation and ingestion. It stores up in the body. Whether inhaled or ingested, fluoride enters the bloodstream.

"Surgeon-General Stewart testified before a U.S. Senate subcommittee on Air Pollution in 1966 that fluorides were pollutants. At the December, 1966

Convention of the American Association for the Advancement of Science, the panelists for the air pollution discussion indicated, in the following order, the most serious air contaminants: sulfur dioxide, ozone, fluorides, chlorine, and ethylene. (*Chem. Week*, Jan. 7, 1967, p. 45.) Dr. Barry Commoner lists fluorides amongst the 'highest priority' pollutants.

"The *New York Times* (Dec. 10, 1963) in an editorial states: 'The most impressive arguments against fluoridation are in fact based not on what we know but on what we do not know. They relate, for example, to what effects fluorides may have within the body. The danger that the accumulation of chemicals can be damaging to health has caused national concern in other connections.'

"Coincidental to this, the *New York Times* of Jan. 10, 1968 reports that the American Dental Association, the arch-proponents of fluoridation, now are warning (after years of unlimited, and untold millions of x-rays of the teeth), that overexposure to x-ray can be lethal or cause birth defects. 'But precisely what constitutes a dangerous radiation dosage has never been determined. Thus, *medical authorities reason that the safest course is to reduce exposure whenever possible.*'

"Why should not this policy of caution be just as truly applicable to fluoridation, the deliberate addition to the public water of an admitted pollutant?"

Very truly yours,
Chester Hardt

The letter illustrates a problem growing progressively more menacing daily. No one can deny that progress carries considerable risk, but substantial proof documented by outstanding scientists, physicians, dentists, biochemists and other distinguished persons demonstrates that fluorides—either in the air or the water—do not represent progress, and that it does not warrant the risk involved.

That risk may be further demonstrated by presenting three cases of death caused or precipitated by fluoride not in the air, but added to drinking water as reported in three leading medical journals.

The first case, reported by Drs. Linsman and McMurray in 1943 in *Radiology* concerned a 22-year-old soldier who was admitted to an Army Hospital in San Antonio for treatment of a stye. This soldier had lived most of his life in 3 Texas cities where water was naturally fluoridated at 1.2 to 5.7 ppm.

An injury to one of his kidneys at 15 years of age had apparently healed, since he was accepted for army service.

While in the hospital routine x-rays showed extensive calcium deposits in his bones, joints and ligaments, especially where the muscles were attached to the bones. He subsequently died from a kidney ailment. Autopsy showed an unusual accumulation of fluoride in his bones, as much as 8,000 ppm. Both kidneys had nearly completely disintegrated. Since research shows that naturally fluoridated water does damage kidneys, a point upon which I shall elaborate in one of the other two cases, it is logical to conclude that fluoride caused his death.

However, if we assume that his injured kidney was overlooked by the examining physician, we then have a weakened kidney that is unable to efficiently eliminate fluoride from the system resulting in fluoride poisoning.

This case points out another fact: the concentration recommended for fluoridation is 1 to 1.2 ppm. If an individual with one damaged kidney died of fluoride poisoning precipitated by drinking water containing fluoride naturally at 1.2 to 5.7 ppm., then there can be no margin of safety.

The second case was that of a 41-year-old nurse who was being treated for a chronic kidney disease with an artificial kidney using fluoridated water in the hemodialysis. This case was reported in the February, 1965 American Medical Association's *Archives of Internal Medicine* by Dr. Taves and collaborators of Rochester, New York.

Hemodialysis is the process of clearing the blood of waste products by withdrawing blood from the body and then returning it after its passage through an "artificial kidney." In this procedure, circulating blood passes through flowing water separated from it by a semipermeable membrane.

In repeated treatments extending over a period

of 8 months, the authors observed that fluoride entered from the water into the bloodstream and settled in the bones instead of the poisonous waste products leaving the blood. Shortly after one of the treatments the patient died in a convulsion contrary to the anticipated improvement from the treatment.

Autopsy showed destructive changes in her bones with an unusually high accumulation of fluoride of about 5,500 ppm. Dr. Singh and others, with many years of fluoride research have reported advanced crippling fluorosis in patients whose bones contained 1,500 ppm. of fluoride.

Except for the period of 1952 to 1957 this nurse drank water that had less than 0.2 ppm. of fluoride. From 1952 to 1957 her home water had approximately 1 ppm. After 1957 she worked in a hospital that had fluoridated water, but she averaged 2 cups of coffee daily. The authors of this paper stated that she retained more fluoride than usual for some time, and that the question of increased retention of fluoride in a patient with kidney disease is not resolved. They attributed the loss of her kidney function to a generalized infection, probably viral, in 1961. Another point is important: Dr. Taves and his associates recommended that hereafter nonfluoridated water be used in these treatments.

A vital statistics report from the *AMA News* just released by the U. S. Department of Health, Education and Welfare states that for most causes of death during 1964, the death rate was lower or about the same as in 1963. Major exceptions, it noted, were kidney infections, up 11 per cent and accidents, up 2 per cent.

The facts just presented make one wonder whether artifically fluoridated water may be responsible for this 11 per cent increase in deaths from kidney infections for the year 1964.

Here are the highlights of another report, this one by Drs. Sauerbrunn, Ryan and Shaw of the Medical and Radiology Services of the VA Hospital in McKinney, Texas and the University of Texas medical school in Dallas.

After a year of invalidism in a nursing home, a 64-year-old man was admitted for the sixth time to the VA Hospital in McKinney, Texas because of severe respiratory distress and semicoma. "At his first hospitalization . . . he complained of pain and of weakness and stiffness of all limbs for several years. He described polydipsia (excessive thirst) and polyuria (passage of unusually large amounts of urine) of at least twenty years' duration, and he had nocturnal incontinence for several months." That had been twelve years before in 1950, which was the first time he was admitted to the VA Hospital. The report went on to describe painstaking blood and urine analyses and x-ray examinations.

"Roentgenograms of the skeleton revealed increased size and density of long bones and of the vertebrae. Calcification of the paravertebral ligaments and calcification of sacrospinous ligaments were noted."

Four years later, in 1954, the same patient was readmitted because of retention of urine and a general inflamed condition. At that time "wasting of muscles of the shoulder girdle was noted for the first time. . . . At this time the patient's neurologic disorder was thought to be caused by spinal cord compression due to extrinsic pressure from an unidentified disease of bone. The polyuria was considered to represent diabetes insipidus.

"Additional admissions in 1955, 1959 and 1961 showed increasing functional urinary obstruction, with repeated urinary tract infection, and progression of crippling skeletal disease." It was determined that the serum levels of calcium, phosphorus and other minerals that might have been involved in the skeletal disorder were actually normal.

"On the final admission (May, 1962) the patient was critically ill with pneumonia and shock, his condition deteriorated rapidly, and he died on the third day after admission."

So here we have a case in which, over a period of twelve years, a patient was admitted to the hospital and intensively studied on six separate occasions, yet the competent and conscientious doctors were not able to correctly diagnose the case until an autopsy was performed after the patient's death. "A toxicologic study disclosed an elevated bone fluoride content of 610 milligrams/100 g. of dried bone and a liver fluoride content of 6.1 milligrams/100 g. of dried liver."

Following up on the question of why this patient should have had such high concentrations of fluoride, the doctors questioned his sister extensively. For most of his life, the patient had drunk well water in areas where the fluoride content of such water is known to be greater than 2 parts per million and less than 3 parts per million. His sister stated that he "always drank excessively large quantities of water and also drank a considerable amount of tea. His diet was unremarkable . . . he rarely consulted a physician, and did not take any self-prescribed medications. He had never had an industrial job." (This ruled out the possibility of occupational fluorosis.) The patient's sister and brother were found to have mottled teeth and the brother had osteoarthritis.

"Drinking water seems to have been his only source of fluoride intake. He appears to have been drinking, for forty-three years, water with concentrations of fluoride from 2.4 ppm. to 3.5 ppm. In the United States these levels of fluoride have not been thought to result in clinically detectable fluorosis except for mottled teeth. This relationship appears to be that for individuals with normal water consumpton. However the risk and degree of fluorosis may also depend on the quantity of water consumed. (Our emphasis.) This corollary is suggested by the findings in our patient who developed severe crippling fluorosis while his brother, who drank the same water, showed only mottling of teeth. The brothers were exposed to identical fluoride concentrations in their drinking water for the same period of time, had the same diet, lived under similar environmental circumstances, but differed by the excessive water intake by our patient."

And these three doctors conclude that prolonged polydipsia—in other words, drinking, for any reason, of considerably more than a quart of water a day that is arbitrarily considered normal—"may be hazardous to persons who live in areas where the levels of fluoride in drinking water are not those usually associated with significant fluorosis."

It may have taken 43 years and heavy drinking of water before this patient wound up in the hospital with chronic fluoride intoxication, eventually to die of it. And it may have taken unusually conscientious doctors determined to find the cause of his death to finally track it down to chronic fluoride intoxication. The case still stands as a demonstration that fluoride does accumulate in the system and that if it is taken long enough, it will eventually do its damage. Let us not forget that there are millions of diabetics, all of whom have an abnormal thirst and probably drink abnormal quantities of water. There are hundreds of thousands of people working in steel mills, other hundreds of thousands sweating in the summer heat on farms, there are heavy coffee drinkers and heavy beer drinkers, and when you add it all up perhaps half of our entire population drinks substantially more water than the four glasses a day that the Public Health Service has decided represent "normal" consumption.

We wonder how many cases similar to this one are showing up in hospitals around the country and *not* being diagnosed as chronic fluoride intoxication because the well-meaning doctors involved don't know what to look for and have been assured so many times that it just can't happen here.

As Louis Lasagna, M.D., the famed Johns Hopkins pharmacologist, put it in a recent article in the *Canadian Medical Association Journal* (July 15, 1967), "My own research suggests that physicians may be affected more by *ex cathedra* textbook statements than by their own clinical experience. Indeed, it is not impossible that a series of inaccurate opinions from a number of distinguished experts could snowball into an overwhelming endorsement or condemnation of a drug."

A fourth case indelibly demonstrates that fluoridated water can be the direct cause of death. This 64-year-old farmer from Texas died on May 13, 1962 at the Veterans Hospital in McKinney, Texas, 3 days after his admission. Follow-up studies of this death were reported by the attending physicians, Drs. Sauerbrunn, Ryan and Shaw in the

December, 1965, issue of the *Annals of Internal Medicine.*

This patient was born and lived in Calhoun, Georgia, where he drank unfluoridated water for the first 7 years of his life. He then moved to Texas where, for 43 years, he drank well water with a concentration of fluoride from 2.4 ppm. to 3.5 ppm. The fact was established that water was the only source of his fluoride intake.

He was first admitted to the Veterans Hospital in McKinney in 1950, at 52 years of age, at which time he complained of pain and cramping of his left leg and weakness and stiffness of arms and legs for several years. He described an excessive thirst with the elimination of large amounts of urine for at least 20 years. The examining physician noted a kyphosis or hunch-back with restriction of spinal movements, stiffness of his knee and ankle joints, spastic weakness of all his extremities and other neurological signs indicative of spinal cord involvement. Tests showed that his kidneys were not eliminating all the waste products from his system. The function of the urinary bladder was impaired with retention of urine.

Two attempts to insert a needle in the spinal canal failed due to the deposition of new bone and calcification of ligaments with loss of normal space between the vertebrae and immobility of the spine.

X-rays showed increased size and density of his long bones and vertebrae. These appeared as marble-white shadows giving the bone a structureless appearance. Ligaments and membranes connecting bones were calcified.

In 1954, the patient was readmitted to the hospital with an increase in the neurological signs of spastic paralysis of all extremities, marked retention of urine and wasting of muscle of the shoulder girdle. X-rays showed increasing bone density.

Additional admissions in 1955, 1959, and 1961 showed increasing functional urinary obstruction, repeated urinary tract infections and progression of his crippling skeleton fluorosis to such an extent that he was confined to a nursing home as a *complete invalid* for one year prior to his death.

An autopsy confirmed the diagnosis of chronic fluoride poisoning.

This case demonstrates that death can occur from chronic fluoride poisoning in an individual exposed to drinking water with less than 4 ppm. of fluoride present as calcium fluoride. It is significant that naturally fluoridated water is about 85 times less toxic than artificially fluoridated water, and natural fluorides are about 1,000 times less soluble than sodium fluoride. This means better elimination and less absorption of fluoride ions.

This patient drank large quantities of water because of excessive thirst. In the opinion of clinical investigators, such as Roholm, fluoride intoxication can cause this marked thirst. The more fluoridated water the individual drinks, the thirstier he becomes.

However, discounting the more than 1 million undetected diabetics who drink 4 to 12 quarts of water daily, there are substantial numbers of people who normally drink 4 to 8 quarts a day—certainly a dangerous dose of fluoride at 1 ppm.

Another important fact to remember is that fluoride poisoning causes such progressive weakness and debilitation that the victim dies from an intercurrent disease as pneumonia.

The history of this case emphasizes another important point: physicians in fluoridated cities may be diagnosing and treating chronic fluoride intoxication as arthritis since these symptoms appear before x-ray evidence of fluorosis.

Chronic fluorosis is difficult to diagnose, even for those doctors who are familiar with it. For those who lack this familiarity and know only that health authorities have assured them that fluoridated water is "non-toxic," there is every reason to believe that such diagnosis is next to impossible.

One of the clearest expositions of the disease-causing potential of fluoride that we have seen comes from the eminent South African scientist, Douw G. Steyn, who is now Chief Research Officer of the Division of Life Sciences of the Atomic Energy Board of South Africa. In September, 1963 Dr. Steyn presented to the Ninth International Convention on Vital Substances, Nutrition and Diseases of Civilization, held in Switzerland and Germany, a full-length discussion of fluoridation and its role in the causation of disease.

He pointed out that fluoride taken internally has two immediate effects: 1. It de-ionizes (neutralizes the electrical charge) calcium present in the blood plasma, thus making it impossible for the calcium to fulfill its metabolic functions; and 2. It poisons important enzyme systems. Dr. Steyn then went on to show how these two biochemical effects lead to a wide variety of disease manifestations. None of these are caused exclusively by fluorine. None of them could be completely eliminated by eliminating fluorine from the diet. But Dr. Steyn and many others have shown that fluorine is one of the causes of each of these diseases, and that it is only reasonable to expect that fluoridation of a city's water will result in sharply increased incidence of each of these ailments.

The following material is all quoted from the above-mentioned presentation by Dr. Steyn in September, 1963. We have deleted from it his many references to the scientific literature which we lack the space to reproduce here.

"Whenever the symptoms of chronic fluorine poisoning are considered, stress is laid on damage done to the normal processes of calcium-phosphorus metabolism (damage to the bones and teeth). Mottling of the teeth is stated to be the earliest symptom of fluorosis. However, once fluorine (fluoride) enters the system (1) it has a strong tendency to combine with calcium thus de-ionising it and rendering it unavailable for many and very important physiological processes in the body, and

(2) it is a very active general enzyme poison. Consequently, it is obvious that many of the initial symptoms of fluorosis are vague and insidious in nature and hence difficult, if not impossible, to diagnose. Fluorine is a poison beset with vagaries and vicissitudes and herein lies its great danger as far as chronic poisoning is concerned. It is clear that before mottling of the teeth, which is a very slow pathologic process, appears, much earlier symptoms of fluorosis due to the deionisation of calcium and to disturbances in enzyme function are bound to be in evidence.

"From the above points it is clear that the earliest detectable clinical symptoms of chronic fluorine poisoning are the result chiefly of deionisation of calcium in the blood and tissues and of disturbances in enzyme action in the body. For these reasons, the following symptoms must be considered in order to obtain an overall picture of fluorosis especially in its incipient stages.

"Calcium is present in cells, in interstitial spaces and in blood serum and plays a very important role in a variety of physiological processes. Normal blood plasma contains 9.0 to 11.0 mg. per cent of calcium; of this amount of calcium only 3.0 to 4.0 mg. per cent is in the ionised form. It is of importance that only the ionised calcium is physiologically active and that only a slight reduction in ionised calcium leads to disturbances of physiological processes in which calcium plays a part. Also of importance is that definite amounts of sodium, potassium, magnesium and calcium are required for their individual ionic balance.

"Excessive amounts of fluoride, beryllium, magnesium or strontium induce bone disorders resembling rickets (Fourman). Fourman states that "Fluoride may produce its effect by inhibiting an enzyme system (Burstone and Keys, 1957). The failure of calcification seems to be associated with a decrease in the amount of ground substance, and hence a decrease in the capacity of the tissue to bind calcium (Belanger, *et al.* 1958).

"Vitamin D does not cure the rickets produced by these foreign ions.

"Hamamoto gives a detailed account of the symptoms of fluorosis in patients as correlated with the fluorine content of their drinking water. Briefly they are: Limitations in the extension and flexion of joints; pains in the back, muscles, joints and limbs; rheumatic pains, stiffness of the limbs, joints, and vertebrae; difficulty in moving about; limited movement of the limbs with swelling. 'In spite of severe bone changes on Roentgenological examination, the general condition of the patients looked rather good.' This has also been our experience with many of the patients in our own investigations in the Republic of South Africa. Also the symptoms described by Hamamoto are in close agreement with those seen by Philip Zanfagna, M.D., in the course of his investigations."

In spite of these dangers, we continue to hear the assurances of public health authorities about the effect of fluoridation on the general health of the population. Not only have no thorough studies ever been made, but even if they were to be made at some time in the future, their accuracy would still depend on the ability of the doctors making the study to recognize chronic fluorosis when they see it.

Do they have the knowledge that will permit them to do this? Not in the opinion of four experts on the subject who have studied it widely in India, publishing a thorough description of chronic fluorosis in the May, 1963 issue of *Medicine,* a bi-monthly medical journal, published by the Williams and Wilkins Company. "Endemic Fluorosis" is the title of the study by Drs. Singh, Jolly, Bansal, and Mather. One of the important points they make is this:

"The dental and skeletal involvements in endemic fluorosis provide the important diagnostic criteria. Dental fluorosis is easily recognized, but the skeletal abnormalities are not so obvious until the advanced stage of crippling fluorosis. However, radiological changes are discernible in the skeleton at a much earlier stage, and provide the only means of diagnosing the early and relatively asymptomatic stage of fluorosis. These cases are young adults whose only complaints are vague pains noted most frequently in the small joints of hands and feet, the knee joints and those of the spine. Such cases are frequent in the endemic area, and may be misdiagnosed as rheumatoid or osteoarthritis. Such symptoms may be present prior to the development of definite radiological signs. A study of the incidence of rheumatic disorders in areas where fluoridation has been in progress for a number of years, would be of interest."

In other words, in the discreet language of doctors who want to make a point without starting a professional feud, these doctors feel there is every possibility that where the water is being fluoridated, people may be developing pains in the joints of their hands and feet, in their knee joints, and in the spine, and that their doctors may be diagnosing these symptoms as rheumatoid arthritis, or osteoarthritis, without the faintest awareness that it is fluorine intoxication that produces them.

In an effort to check on this hypothesis—that doctors in fluoridated cities may be diagnosing and treating chronic fluorine intoxication as arthritis—we have attempted to obtain comparable figures on the incidence of rheumatoid and osteoarthritis in such long-fluoridated cities as Newburgh, New York; Grand Rapids, Michigan; and Philadelphia, Pennsylvania. No figures are available, we have been informed. Since arthritis only cripples you, but does not kill you and is not contagious, doctors are not required to report their cases to the health authorities. Nobody can say with accuracy whether ailments diagnosed as the arthritic diseases are on the increase in fluoridated areas. In fact, since arthritis is a bone disease, whose cause is unknown, and which takes its greatest toll of heavy water drinkers—farmers and factory workers—we doubt whether anyone can say with certainty that arthritis is not related to fluoride intake. At least, the two so closely resemble each other that it is an easy matter for a doctor, familiar with arthritis, but assured by the Public Health Service that there is no such thing as intoxication from fluoride consumed at the level of one part per million, to mistake the one for the other. Until the Public Health Service gets around to making a study of what has happened to the rate of incidence of arthritic diseases in fluoridated cities, its assurances of safety are obviously more a matter of opinion than of hard scientific fact.

Symptoms of Fluorosis

Here then, for the benefit of doctors who ought to know how to recognize the subtle poisoning, and those of the public who will yet vote on the issue of whether or not to adopt water fluoridation, are the symptoms of chronic fluorine intoxication as they were learned by four Indian doctors in studying 409 cases over a period of seven years, and reporting their study in *Medicine.*

1. Mottling of the tooth enamel is considered by these doctors to have a great deal more than merely "aesthetic significance." They state that "this mottling of enamel is one of the first and earliest visible signs of an excessive intake of fluorine

in early childhood. It is usually regarded as a suggestive diagnostic criterion, and has been accepted as an index of fluorosis." In other words, the 20 per cent of the children in fluoridated cities who develop mottled enamel, may be assumed to be suffering from a general fluorosis, and not merely from discoloration of their teeth.

2. Skeletal examination revealed great changes in the spine, particularly in the cervical region. "The vertebrae showed altered proportions and measurements in all planes, but the striking abnormality was the gross reduction of the antero-posterior diameter of the spinal canal which, in the case studied at autopsy, was reduced to 2 mm. at the level of third and fourth cervical vertebrae. Since the average antero-posterior diameter of the spinal cord in the cervical enlargement is 8 mm., and the bulge of the ligamentum flavum has to be accommodated, it is evident that compression of the cord is almost inevitable."

This discovery is a highly significant one. Fluoride has been found to lead to the deposition of new bone within the spinal canal. This causes constriction of the spinal cord, the obvious cause of one terrifying end result these doctors have found —that chronic fluorosis can lead to paraplegia.

3. "The irregular bone deposition was obvious clinically in a large percentage of cases as bony excrescences of varying size. These were usually seen near the knee joint, along the anterior border of the tibia, and near the olecranon . . . 86 of our

cases had crippling deformities due partly to mechanical dysfunction, and partly to immobilization necessitated by pain."

This is the kind of condition, visible in x-ray, that many doctors will tend to diagnose as arthritis.

4. Osteosclerosis, an increase in the weight and density of bone, which can sometimes result in spontaneous fractures, was observed in the spine and the pelvis.

5. In 42 of the 409 cases, there were neurological complications. The authors speculate that the symptoms may be due to the involvement of the spinal cord, or a lesion of one or more nerve roots. "The most important manifestations were muscular wasting, acro-paresthesiae (abnormal sensations in the hands and feet), and pain, which were almost universally present. . . . The most important feature was the weakness and wasting of muscles. This was usually asymmetrical, involving most often the small muscles of one or both hands.

"The earliest symptom of spinal cord involvement, present in all cases, was weakness of both lower limbs. This usually started in one leg, with later progression to the other. In 18 cases, after a variable interval, the upper limbs became involved, producing a spastic quadriplegia. . . . The pattern resembled in many ways that of spondylitic myelopathy . . ." (inflammation of the nerve sheath of the spine). It is pointed out that, in addition to arthritis, fluorosis may closely simulate spinal inflammations and tumors.

The authors point out that fluorosis is not easy to recognize in its early stages. Sometimes there are changes discernible by x-ray before there are any complaints from the patient. At other times there may be complaints of vague pains in the joints and spine before any changes may be seen by radiology. "The dental and skeletal involvement in endemic fluorosis provide the important diagnostic criteria. Dental fluorosis is easily recognized, but the skeletal abnormalities are not so obvious until the advanced stage of crippling fluorosis." Therefore, to add our own comment, the importance of dental fluorosis must never be under-estimated. If there is mottling of the teeth, there is a general intoxication of the system which is ultimately going to lead to far more serious results.

Not to unduly alarm our readers, let us point out that this Indian study was made in a region where most (though not all) of the water has a natural fluoride concentration considerably above the one part per million that is recommended by the Public Health Service. This study alone does not prove that a concentration of one part per million of fluoride in the water will have the same dreadful results. Our basic point is that it has never been proven that a concentration of one ppm. will not have these same results of fluorosis.

We know that this low concentration causes dental fluorosis in 20 per cent of the children who drink it. And it has been pointed out that dental fluorosis is the earliest and most reliable diagnostic sign of more terrible complications to come. Nobody has ever taken the trouble to make a thorough study of the ultimate results of a lifetime of drinking water fluoridated at one ppm.

Nor has anyone taken the time to do a scientific study on the dangers of fluoride in the air. It's high time we learned some answers. Without them, who's to guarantee how much longer we'll be around to ask questions?

CHAPTER XII

Rheumatism—What Is It?

IN THE early chapters of this book, we pointed out that rheumatism, unlike arthritis, is a virtually meaningless term. It should never have been allowed to find its way into medical nomenclature, and, in fact, no doctor will use the word when talking to fellow physicians. But the average man does go on using it, and to him it is a general term indicating a disease of the muscles, tendons, joints, bones, nerves—virtually any ache or pain is referred to by the man on the street as rheumatism. When asked whether he thinks he's suffering from arthritis or rheumatism, he will be hard put to answer—and there is no wonder. For, according to this general popular definition, arthritis is one form of rheumatism. Other forms include bursitis, neuritis, lumbago, sciatica, and gout, among many, many others.

Recently, a somewhat better definition of rheumatism has been offered which includes all diseases of the musculo-skeletal structure other than those involving the joints, exclusively. Yet, it is generally agreed by those in the field that a more uniform and clear-cut definition of the rheumatic diseases is sorely needed.

But if a definition of rheumatism seems elusive, the causes and treatment of the many diseases lumped together under the title "rheumatism" are far more so. Some authorities, for example, believe that a predisposition to rheumatoid diseases is inherited. Certain drugs bring about specific rheumatoid diseases, as do metabolic imbalances in the body, excessive stress and countless other factors.

For example, the rheumatic disease systemic lupus erythematosus may be related to drugs, according to John J. Sampson, M.D. and three Medical Corps associates. In an article in the *Journal of the American Medical Association* (May 10, 1965, Vol. 192, No. 6), they note, "an increasing number of drugs have been implicated in the development of systemic lupus erythematosus."

For victims of SLE (a degenerative disease of the blood cells and tissues), there is an almost endless variety or combination of symptoms. On the cheeks, neck and chest, disk-like patches usually appear. These characteristic patches have raised, reddish edges and are covered with scales and crusts. Besides skin damage, the *Merck Manual*

(Merck and Co., Inc., 1961) says a typical SLE case includes: fever, joint pains, kidney inflammation, an abnormally high globulin content of the blood, and a reduction in the number of leukocytes (colorless corpuscles) in the blood. Although lesions are especially common in the skin, spleen and kidneys, the *Manual* says "any tissue may show involvement."

The consequences SLE presents offer extremely dangerous alternatives. Either the acute disease will be fatal within a few weeks, or the disease may run a chronic remittent course, causing semi-invalidism for years. An article in *Public Health Reports* (Vol. 77, No. 9, September, 1962) informs us that 80 per cent of SLE victims may suffer from anemia; 90 per cent from inflammation of the joints (often indistinguishable from rheumatoid arthritis); and more than 50 per cent are victims of pleurisy (often resembling pneumonia and frequently complicated by infection). That's not all—SLE-caused nervous system disorders include fits, hallucinations, and paranoia.

Alarmingly enough, the *Merck Manual* states that for "reasons unknown," SLE has become "more prevalent in recent years." One explanation for the rise in cases may be the increasing use of anti-convulsant drugs—the drugs most frequently implicated as inducers of SLE.

Two of these drugs are pointed out by Dr. Howard L. Holley, Chief of the Rheumatology Section of the University of Alabama Medical Center.

In his study, four children with convulsive disorders were examined. During the period in which these children suffered seizures (three to eight years), their therapy consisted principally of the drugs Trimethadione and Diphenylhydantoin. Dr. Holley reported (*Arthritis and Rheumatism,* Vol. 7, No. 6, December, 1964) that while undergoing this drug treatment, every child developed SLE.

In an earlier study, investigators found 18 patients who developed SLE after long-term chemotherapy. According to *Medical Tribune's* report (June 28, 1963) treatment was for unrelated diseases—epilepsy, hypertension and tuberculosis. One of the investigators and Director of Maimonides Hospital's Division of Hematology, Dr. Stanley L. Lee, said that although a number of the patients had been taking more than one drug, in three cases diphenylhydantoin was the only drug administered.

No matter how you look at it, these drugs are a risky form of therapy. While exactly how anticonvulsant drugs induce SLE remains unknown, Dr. Holley believes they could possibly be the "trigger mechanism" that initiates a reaction. One thing is certain—the problem they present is extremely serious. As the use of these drugs grows increasingly common, so may not only SLE but other rheumatic diseases as well.

But to lay the cause of all forms of rheumatism at the doorstep of drug therapy would be hopelessly oversimplifying and totally false. Even SLE must be the result of factors other than drugs in a good many cases. But the point is this: Whereas the other factors have not yet been found and so cannot be conscientiously avoided, one factor—the drugs we have discussed—has been identified and *can* be avoided.

Another factor that has been recognized to play a part in the development of certain rheumatoid diseases is dietary imbalance or deficiency. We will discuss this at great length in relation to important specific diseases in further chapters. But let's point out some examples here.

Considerable investigation has been carried out on the subject of vitamin E and rheumatism. C. L. Steinberg, M.D., told in the *Annals of the New York Academy of Science* for October 3, 1949, of his success in giving vitamin E to rheumatic patients. Treating fibrositis (muscular rheumatism) in 300 patients with vitamin E, he found that relief was obtained in the vast majority of cases. He cautions that the patient should keep on taking a "maintenance" dose, after the symptoms have disappeared.

He also treated rheumatic fever with vitamin E. He relates five case histories of young people whose rheumatic fever symptoms were relieved by vitamin E. It is interesting to note that he gave natural (not synthetic) vitamin E throughout the experiment.

Dr. Morris Ant of Kings County Hospital, Brooklyn, treats muscle diseases and industrial injuries with wheat germ oil directly applied to the painful spot. Reporting on his experiences in *Industrial Medicine* for June, 1946, he tells us he used a 55 per cent ointment of wheat germ oil and food supplementation by wheat germ oil, as well as a diet rich in vitamin E foods. Out of 20 cases treated successfully, he reports in detail on four—one a housewife whose hands were swollen and stiff. Local application of wheat germ oil soon returned the hands to their normal condition. A physician with swelling of his knees and back so painful that he could not walk was given wheat germ oil locally and internally and was soon able to resume his practice once more. An elevator operator who had had a serious fall developed pain and stiff muscles in his chest and legs along with bronchial asthma. After several months of wheat germ oil therapy both locally and internally he went back to work free from all symptoms except for a slight occasional limp. Incidentally the asthma disappeared, too. A clerk who had fallen against the sharp corner of a desk suffered from a long-standing pain over her ribs, so violent that she was unable to sleep. Wheat germ oil locally and internally left her symptom-free within months.

In a later article in *The Annals of the New York Academy of Science* Dr. Ant, along with Erwin Di-Cyan describes the use of vitamin E in rheumatic diseases—this time given orally, intramuscularly and locally. In a series of 100 patients, there was relief from pain, improvement or disappearance of physical symptoms and increased mobility of joints. In addition to the therapy which these patients received at the doctor's office they were placed on diets high in vitamin E—for instance, a tablespoon of wheat germ was taken at breakfast, one-fourth head of lettuce with peanut oil dressing and one banana were added to the lunch menu. A dinner of lean beef, spinach and lettuce with peanut oil dressing contributed to the vitamin E content of the day's meal.

C. L. Steinberg was not the only one to feel that diet played a role in the development of rheumatic fever. He treated the disease with vitamin E, but a number of physicians have reported success in treating it with eggs. An editorial in the *British Medical Journal* for April 17, 1954 discusses the subject at length. May G. Wilson in a book, *Rheumatic Fever,* published by Oxford University Press, 1940, speculates on the fact that cases of rheumatic fever reach their peak in April and then decline during the summer months. Eggs are plentiful and hence cheap during spring and summer, scarce and hence expensive during winter. Could the eating of eggs be related therefore to the incidence of rheumatic fever?

The reasoning goes like this: eggs are rich in a B vitamin, choline. This vitamin is extremely important for the health of the liver. It helps to manufacture a substance called phosopholipid a fatty substance for the blood. This substance is one of the elements that fights against streptococcus infection. Rheumatic fever is associated with streptococcus infection. Therefore, rheumatic fever may be conditioned partly at least by egg intake.

Wallis, writing in the *American Journal of Medical Science,* volume 227, page 167, 1954 states that he did a survey among 184 adult and adolescent patients with rheumatic heart disease and a group of normal subjects. Forty-one per cent of the rheumatic heart patients said they thought they ate few eggs in childhood. Only 16 per cent of the normal people claimed they did not eat eggs as children. Ten per cent of the rheumatic patients said they still did not like eggs; only five per cent of the healthy folks had this food prejudice.

You may say that such a survey could not be significant enough to base a theory on, since it depends on the patients' memories of what they ate as children. However, rather elaborate precautions were taken during the survey to eliminate any biased answers.

Two other researchers, Coburn and Moore, reporting in the *American Journal of Diseases of Children,* volume 65, page 744, 1943 state that the diet of rheumatic heart children appeared to be lacking in eggs as well as other valuable nutritional elements. So they supplemented the diet of 30 convalescent children with the equivalent of four egg yolks a day (the yolk of the eggs is the part highest in choline and other fats). The rheumatic fever recurred in only seven per cent of these children compared with a recurrence of 38 per cent in children whose diets were not so supplemented. Later in 1950 Dr. Coburn reported in the *Journal of the American Dietetic Association,* volume 26, page 345, that eight to ten egg yolks daily given to children who had previously had rheumatic fever prevented relapses even when the children were later subjected to streptococcal infection.

Now we have uncovered another piece of evidence implicating eggless diets as possible predisposing causes of rheumatic fever. Dr. Coburn and two colleagues writing in *The Journal of Experimental Medicine,* volume 100, page 425, 1954, tell us of experiments in which they induced rheumatism in laboratory animals by eliminating eggs and prevented it by giving egg yolks. Here, surely, is another link in the chain of evidence that will one day lead to the complete elimination of this disease.

The authors tell us their experiments show that under certain conditions, "some lipid substance," that is, some fatty substance, of egg yolk will prevent the animal from getting rheumatic symptoms when a substance is given him that would otherwise produce them. Now, note carefully the following further observations: it did no good to give the egg yolk daily to adult animals which were at the same time subjected to the rheumatism-producing substance. But animals born and bred throughout their lifetimes on diets which included egg yolk received a high degree of protection when they were later subjected to conditions that would have caused rheumatism. Supplementing the diet with egg yolk even two to four weeks before inducing the disease gave some protection.

The authors go on to say "Attention is called to the possibility that these experimental findings . . . (on arthritis) may be pertinent to the genesis of the rheumatic state." The factors among "less privileged" persons which favor the development of rheumatic fever are not well defined. In other words, we do not know exactly what kind of diet is eaten generally by children who later come down with rheumatic fever. But there seems to be no doubt that it is lacking in natural fatty substances. Rheumatic fever does not occur in patients who have a high level of fat in the blood (diabetics, for instance) but it does occur in cases of Graves's disease where the blood level of fat is low.

What was the substance in egg yolk that gave the protection? The authors do not know. But they do know that it was a fatty substance. And they found, too, that breaking down crude lecithin gave them a substance which protected the animals against the rheumatism.

We hear a lot of frightening facts about fats in the diet these days. Headlines in newspapers and magazines caution us against eating eggs because, we are told, eggs contain cholesterol and cholesterol seems to be responsible for the fatty deposits that cause hardening of the arteries. Sure, eggs contain cholesterol, but they also contain lecithin which, scientific research indicates, emulsifies cholesterol so that it does not collect where it is not wanted. Hence the cholesterol content of eggs cannot harm you, because it comes equipped with the one substance that (in nature) controls and directs it.

Do the children in your family like eggs? If the adults not only eat eggs but exclaim about how delicious they are, chances are the young ones will do the same. An egg a day is a passport to vitamin A, D and E, lots of good minerals, especially iron to prevent anemia, and plenty of all the B vitamins, even the most obscure ones. As we have seen above, eggs also contain some kind of fatty substance (can it be lecithin or something else?) that protects against rheumatic tendencies.

To show just how important diet can be in treating some forms of rheumatism, we'll close this chapter with a discussion of an article by Dorothy C. Hare, C.B.E., M.D., published in the British journal *Proceedings of the Royal Society of Medicine,* Vol. 30, 1936. Dr. Hare contributes what seems to be the most convincing piece of evidence on diet influencing the course of chronic rheumatism. Dr. Hare describes an experiment at the Royal Free Hospital in which rheumatic patients received a diet of raw fruits and vegetables with results that were, it seems to us, spectacular. Dr. Hare is apparently a conservative physician who indicates that she does not advise this diet to replace other forms of medical therapy nor does she advise it in all cases. She simply reports on it and suggests that further research would be valuable.

Twelve patients were selected for the experiment—all were sent to the hospital for this purpose. They represented the main types of rheumatism, as well as osteoarthritis and rheumatoid arthritis. No other treatment was given them aside from the diet; they were encouraged to be up and around, whenever the severity of their ailment allowed. Some of them were bedridden.

After they became accustomed to the hospital life, eating the diet usually served in the wards for one week, they were placed for two weeks on a diet consisting of nothing but fresh, raw fruits and vegetables, nuts, cream, salad oil, milk and raw oatmeal.

A day's menu went like this:

Breakfast—apple porridge made of grated apple, soaked raw oatmeal, grated nuts, cream, fresh orange, tea with milk and cream.

Mid-Morning—tomato puree with lemon.

Dinner—salad of lettuce, cabbage, tomato, root vegetables
salad dressing with oil
mixed fruit salad and cream

Tea—dried fruits, nuts and tea with milk and cream.

Supper—fruit porridge, prune, apricot or apple salad dish with dressing.

Bedtime—lemon and orange juice with hot water.

After two weeks, the following cooked foods were added to this diet:

vegetable soup	two ounces of bacon
one egg	two ounces of bread
two ounces of meat	butter, cheese and milk

At no time during the weeks of the diet was any salt added to either the raw or cooked foods. The dried fruits and raw oatmeal were soaked in water, the vegetables were shredded, nuts crushed or whole. All food was prepared fresh for every meal and was served attractively.

Eight of the patients began to feel better in one to four weeks on this diet. Two improved up to 5 or 6 weeks, then relapsed. Two showed no improvement at all. In the follow-up, after the patients who improved had gone home, it was found that 7 of them continued to improve to a marked degree. For example, one patient aged 46 had suffered for 4 years with occasional pain and swelling of the knees, but for the 3 months before she was admitted to the hospital, she had general pain and stiffness in shoulders, arms, hands, knees, and legs. She had been in bed for 10 weeks. There was fluid in both knee joints, swelling and pain in other joints. She was discharged from the hospital after being on the diet for 3 weeks. Later, after continuing with the diet for 7 more weeks, she was free from all pain and able to do her housework.

All of the patients lost considerable weight during the first week on the diet, but those who continued to lose in the following weeks lost much less, and in every case except very obese patients weight was properly maintained on the diet. For the obese patients, of course, losing weight was extremely helpful, as overweight adds greatly to the problems of those suffering from rheumatism and arthritis.

In commenting on her diet and its success, Dr. Hare remarks on the fact that the rawness of the food seemed to be the one outstanding factor that brought about results. The fact that the food was raw made a great impression on the patients themselves and on observers. She tells us that a Zurich physician who used raw diets similar to this in treating rheumatism claimed that the diet was successful "because of the absorption of the unaltered solar energy of plant life." Says Dr. Hare "science has so far revealed nothing . . . of this occult solar energy, as something apart from vitamin and chemical constituents (of food)."

We have made no study of "occult solar energy" but it seems that science will soon have to be convinced of the healthfulness of raw foods, for every day we are finding out more and more about the vitamins and enzymes destroyed by heating foods. May there not be many other elements in food, unknown as yet to science, that we destroy when the food is heated above body temperature?

Then, says Dr. Hare, such a diet contains a lot of vitamin C and B (as well as A, we can add). Protein and fat are lacking in the vegetables and fruits. This deficiency is partly made up for by the cream, nuts, and salad oil, later by the meat, eggs and cheese. Finally, Dr. Hare remarks, we must consider how much of the effectiveness of the diet depends on the fact that it was low in sodium. Vegetables contain little sodium and considerable potassium. No salt (sodium chloride) was added at any time during the diet, so that, even though bacon and other foods were added later on, the diet was still extremely low in sodium compared to the usual diet.

So far we have been talking about rheumatism in a general way. In the following chapters we will discuss specific diseases and ailments, what some researchers think causes them, and what can be done to alleviate the suffering and often cure the disease itself.

CHAPTER XIII

Neuritis

ONE OF THE most prevalent of all rheumatic diseases—as well as one of the most painful—is neuritis. Neuritis, according to the *American College Dictionary*, is the inflammation of a nerve. More to the point, especially to the neuritis sufferer, is that the disease produces continuous pain in the nerve either because the nerve is being irritated or because it is itself diseased.

Neuritis can occur anywhere in the body, since nerve endings occur by the millions almost everywhere, from scalp to toes. Sciatica, pain along the sciatic nerve, is normally a type of neuritis. We will deal with sciatica in a separate chapter. But most often, the disease attacks the hands, arms, shoulders and neck region. Most attacks occur in the shoulders, and are so common they have come to be designated as "painful shoulder," in medical jargon as a synonym for neuritis of the shoulder.

Mark B. Coventry, M.D., of Mayo Clinic in Rochester, Minnesota, discusses painful shoulder in an article in the *Journal of the American Medical Association,* January 17, 1953. He says there are 4 possible causes: 1. muscular—which may mean overuse, fractures, dislocations, bad posture, tumors or calcification of joints; 2. nervous—caused by inflammation of nerves; 3. visceral—that is, the shoulder pain may actually originate in a gall bladder, heart or pancreas disorder; and 4. vascular—when there is a disorder of the blood vessels.

He discusses the possibility of occupational causes for shoulder pain. One patient of his worked in an overall factory, and when he had finished his particular operation on a pair of heavy overalls, he had to throw them over his shoulder onto a pile. Shoulder pain is also common among farmers after a session of especially heavy work such as silo-filling. But some occupational hazards are less obvious. One of Dr. Coventry's patients was a retired school teacher who had taken a job as a typist. The extended position of her arms as she typed all day was the cause of her painful shoulder. Another patient was a baker who decorated cakes. Apparently he stooped over a table, with his muscles tense, all day as he worked away at this very fine and intricate work.

Disuse can cause a painful or stiff shoulder, says Dr. Coventry. When a joint has been immobilized in a cast, of course there is pain when you begin to use it again. On the other hand, when there is pain, you have a tendency not to use the shoulder, so that it becomes stiff. Then when you try to use it again, those creaking unused muscles give you such a twinge that you decide not to try to use them, thus leading to more stiffness.

Finally, says Dr. Coventry, there is the factor of the "personality." A painful shoulder becomes stiff only if the patient does not use it and if the patient has a personality which makes him susceptible to this kind of disorder.

Three physicians of Madison, Wisconsin, discuss this kind of personality in greater detail in an article in the *American Practitioner* for May, 1953. They examined 300 patients who seemed to have psychosomatic illnesses and found that 60 of them suffered from pain and stiffness in the shoulder. Their ages ranged from 25 to 55 years; most of them were in their forties. The majority of them had other complaints along with their bad shoulders: headaches, some kind of chronic nose trouble, weakness and fatigue, dizzy spells, stomach trouble, heart trouble or some muscular discomfort, such as muscular aches, cramps in the legs and so forth. All of them, say our physicians, were tense and likely to overreact to physical stimulus—the kind of people who jump nervously at a hand laid on the shoulder or a leaf dropped on the hand. In most of these folks, an x-ray showed no physical injury or disorder in the shoulder.

Questioning elicited the discovery that in almost all cases the pain and stiffness had begun at a time of particular stress and heightened emotion. This does not mean necessarily some grave emergency. These people were the perfectionist kind who thought of themselves as self-sufficient, independent and energetic. They were all overly conscientious. They lived well-planned lives, following rigid patterns of activity and any interruption of their well-laid plans brought frustration. But, gritting their teeth, they "carried on" bravely, all the time unconsciously resenting the fact that their responsibilities were too heavy.

In their daily work they did not use their hands or arms more than the average person, but they did everything with their muscles under tension which created a lot of resistance in the voluntary muscles which were working along at their usual speed and tension. "The protracted co-existence of these two opposing forces plus the vulnerability of the shoulder joint might explain why this structure is so frequently the site of this type of musculoskeletal disability," say the authors.

So these patients were given psychotherapy. We do not know of what this consisted. But we suppose that the psychiatrist or psychologist simply by talking to them managed to convince them that there was absolutely no need to be so tense, hurried and conscientious about the things they were doing. Actually no matter how hard we try none of us can be perfect. So if we plan to get something done by noon, let's try working at it in a relaxed fashion. If we succeed, fine. If not, then let's not get worried, tense and upset about it. Let's postpone it for the next day, without any regrets or self-blame. This is not a plea for laziness. But those folks who work (or play) at too intense a pitch are well aware of what they are doing. And if they wish to avoid ill health, they simply must learn to relax and not try so hard for perfection. In the case of the 60 patients, the psychotherapy worked wonders. They learned to take things much easier and, as their muscles relaxed, their shoulder pain disappeared.

All the articles in our file on painful shoulder mention the factor of personality. Whether you take it from the point of view of a psychosomatic personality—that is, someone who unconsciously interprets frustration or insecurity in terms of actual physical illness—or whether you decide that the muscular strain of such overly conscientious people results in stiffness and pain in the shoulder, it boils down to the same thing—a defect in personality that somehow brings about a quite serious and common disorder.

Common methods of cure include various pain-killing drugs, deep x-ray, diathermy, injections of novocaine and posture exercises. Of these, we can only recommend posture exercises. Our field is not cure, but it seems to us that painful shoulder might be prevented by sensible rules of good health. We all know surely when we are overworking some particular part of us, and we should know enough to stop before this overwork results in pain or stiffness. Yes, even if it means changing jobs, it would certainly be worth it.

Our research has shown us, too, that vitamin B and calcium are preventatives of muscle stiffness. The diets of most of us are deficient in these two food elements. Brewer's yeast and bone meal are good sources.

Several years ago J. I. Rodale noticed that his right shoulder was painful. He thought it might come from doing so much writing with a pencil gripped hard in his hand. He switched to a typewriter and the pain disappeared. But he did not like to type, so he had to find some other solution. He began to use his left hand, rather than his right, whenever he could—in opening doors, putting on his hat, eating, brushing his hair and so forth. As he gradually began to make his left hand do more of the inconsequential manual work, his right shoulder improved. Furthermore, he did a little research and found that the theory of using one side to rest the other side has long been known to primitive people. The American Indians practiced it in their long journeys by land. They marched part of the way using the right foot harder than the left, then shifted and made the left foot do more work.

Interestingly enough, time and motion study experts, whose profession it is to get industrial jobs done with the least effort, the most production and the greatest saving of time, have found that one of their most important principles is to get both hands to share the work, so that neither of them becomes overly tired. Time and again, by proper planning, these experts have arranged a given piece of work so that both hands work at once or so that each hand works equally with the other, thus saving time, motion, money—and incidentally, making the job faster, easier and not so tiring for the worker.

One final caution. It seems to us quite possible that an explanation of many of the cases of stiff shoulder which become worse at night might very well be incorrect sleeping positions assumed. J. I. Rodale has covered the subject thoroughly in his book *Sleep and Rheumatism.* In the following pages are some important selections from that book:

"I would like to tell you the story of how I stumbled upon an interesting fact about neuritis.

"Around 1940 I began to experience neuritic pains in the hands, arms and shoulders. There would be dull twinges and pains, and I found it extremely difficult to don my overcoat. If I raised my arms above a certain level the pain would increase. I couldn't turn my head without experiencing pain in the neck and shoulders. I would get up in the morning with a feeling in the shoulders and neck as if someone had sat on me all night, and my fingers had a numbness which made it difficult for me to tie my shoelaces.

"The doctor diagnosed it as neuritis, but its cause had him baffled, and in spite of months of medical treatments of all kinds, including osteopathy the painful condition persisted. As I look back now I can see that in this doctor's practice, he specialized in finding cures, but never spent any time in seeking causes. He asked me no questions about my daily life and habits in order to come upon some clue that might lead to the answer. I just kept coming and he kept treating it, mainly with diathermy, but nothing happened.

"A friend of mine had about the same symptoms that I did and every time we would meet we would swap talk about our condition.

"One night I discovered the cause of my trouble. It was about 3:00 a.m. when I suddenly awoke from a disturbed sleep. My entire arm was numb from shoulder to finger tips. In fact it was practically paralyzed. I tried to think quickly, and noticed that I had been sleeping with my head on the paralyzed arm. I became convinced that this habit was at the bottom of all my trouble. My own hard head had been digging down on my arm for hours.

"I stayed awake for a long time thinking, and observing the actions of my arms and head. I would catch my arm attempting to move upward so that it could be a pillow to my head, but I fought against it. It took about a week to win complete control over them, and after that the habit was completely mastered. Never again did I sleep with my head on my arms, and miracle of miracles, the neuritis in my arms completely vanished.

"I then went to see my friend who had the same condition I did, and when I related my experience to him, a light came into his eyes. He did not sleep with his head on his arms. In his case it was a way he had of folding back his left arm in a v-shape and sleeping with his body pressing on it. He now cured himself of this habit, sleeping with his arm spread out in a relaxed way, and within a week his neuritic pains completely disappeared.

"When I saw how simple it was to cure these two cases I began to think of the hundreds of thousands of people who must be suffering from the same thing, and since in questioning people I found that a majority of them did sleep with their head pressing on their arms, I figured that I had a job to do. I had to share my knowledge with as many persons as possible. So I wrote a book on the subject in 1940, as well as several articles which appeared at that time in *Fact Digest* and *True Health Stories,* two magazines which I edited and owned. As a result hundreds of people have been cured of what I call pressure neuritis.

"I was surprised when in 1944, Dr. Robert Wartenberg sent me a reprint of an article he wrote in the *Journal of Nervous and Mental Disease* (May, 1944), in which he mentioned my work in this field. I was surprised that a physician would mention the work of a layman.

"A doctor friend of mine, a phlebitis specialist in New York, was incensed when he received a copy of my book, and said to me at our next meeting, Why do you meddle in such things? You are not a doctor.

"To give you another reaction from a doctor, may I quote from a letter received from Mrs. Susan Snyder, 135 Eastern Parkway, Brooklyn, N.Y. (Oct. 29, 1953):

"The doctor tells me that I have osteoarthritis. The pains I complained about—terrific headaches and pains from the back of the neck up and down to lower back as well as between shoulders completely disappeared after I arose and walked about for about a half hour. I asked my doctor (an M.D.) if it wasn't pressure pains. I suspected what your book confirmed. The doctor gave me some 'double talk' and said that the pain was due to adhesions, and he suggested 'radar' treatments. I went three times a week until your book opened my eyes. I was mad clean through. Why wasn't my doctor honest enough to tell me that the pains were due to pressure exerted in sleep?

"I sent him your book and told him 'I know and so does Mr. Rodale that osteoarthritis is incurable (degenerated bones cannot be restored) but I am glad to have been corroborated in my suspicion that my pains were pressure pains and I didn't need a doctor for that.'"

"Mrs. Snyder turned over to me the answer from her physician. He said, 'Proper sleeping habits are helpful in these conditions—but by no means curative—since they do not remove the, as yet, unknown cause or causes. Mr. Rodale oversimplifies the entire matter principally through ignorance of the basic sciences relating to the human body. Improvement by any method of treatment may be only apparent, concurrent and coincident with a period of natural remission of symptoms—which usually recur in spite of the continuance of the temporarily "miraculous cure".'

"I make no comment except to say that my own cure has so far been in effect for over 16 years. Many others have had similar experiences. I have had hundreds of letters testifying to my method's efficaciousness in completely clearing up pressure neuritis.

"Here is a typical case: One day I was in a broker's office and overheard the bookkeeper complaining to a customer's man that she had been having terrible pains in her arms and shoulders. I have to go to my doctor this afternoon for vitamin B injections and I dread going, she said. And tomorrow I am supposed to go to my dentist to have my teeth x-rayed. The doctor thinks that it might be infected teeth, and I might have to have all of them extracted.

"I walked over to her and related my own experience. When I explained that possibly head pressure could be the cause of her own trouble she was delighted to find an excuse for not going to the doctor or dentist. She at once admitted that she slept with her head on her arms. In about a week that girl was as free of pain as a new-born baby, without the benefit of any vitamin B injections. Of course not everyone who has pains in the arms and shoulders gets them from sleep pressures, but it is surprising how many cases do arise from this cause.

"Here are a few letters received from readers who have benefited from my book on the subject. They are only a few chosen from hundreds:

"Here is one from Bernard Singer, 16 Shanley Ave., Newark, N.J.:

"I had been experiencing sharp pains across the back occasionally. After reading your pamphlet I became aware of two faulty sleeping habits. I was resting my head on my right arm and my wife threw one leg frequently over my back as I slept. By avoiding these two faulty habits, I have found that my backaches disappeared."

"James M. Moore, Route 4, Greenville, Ohio writes:

"I had found my two big toes were becoming numb, with almost no feeling in them. By breaking myself of lying so that one leg was under the other, this situation has cleared up also. Now these toes have a normal feeling."

"Mrs. C. C. Wacker, Wilton Junction, Iowa writes:

"I used to wake up more tired than when I went to bed, and so full of aches and pains that I was miserable—until I read your book *Sleep and Rheumatism.* Now I wake up refreshed. It's almost like a miracle. Others have been helped by your method through my telling them, including my husband who has been greatly benefitted. So we decided to give four of these books as Christmas presents."

"John H. Stevenson, 26 Southbridge St., Worcester, Massachusetts writes:

"Your book *Sleep and Rheumatism* has taught me how to get more rest in my sleeping hours. Now I get up in the morning without that swollen feeling in my hands, which our family doctor says is a sign of arthritis. We are hearing too much about that dreadful trouble, and I believe you have told me how to stop it."

"Hugo Mayerhoefer, Salem, Oregon:

"My dear Mr. Rodale: Your book *Sleep and Rheumatism* told me exactly where 90 per cent of my rheumatism came from. However, none of the positions you illustrated fit my case and so it did no good for about a year or so until I finally discovered that my collarbone, in sleeping on my side, pressed against some nerve and choked off the supply line and a few weeks after noticed a change for the better. Twenty years suffering because my doctors didn't find the cause of my trouble. A million thanks to you."

"The sleep neuritis comes from pressure on nerves which damages them, and also from blood congestions caused by pressure on veins, but the amazing thing is how quickly the condition clears up when the sleep pressures are eliminated. You might ask, but how can I prevent myself from doing these things during sleep? The answer is that you begin by trying, and pretty soon your subconscious mind has learned a new set of sleeping habits. All you need do is draw an imaginary line along your shoulders, and in sleep never let your arms go above that line, and keep your arms down at the sides, and as relaxed as possible.

"In Germany, a survey made a few years ago showed that practically 100 per cent of the population aged between 40 and 50 were afflicted with some form of arthritis or neuritis, but this of course included very mild cases. Ask any person over 60 and you will find that they are suffering from vague bodily pains and twinges. Many of these cases are due to pressures exerted in sleep, although I have also found that some of it is due to sleeping on soft mattresses, which cause the spine to curve downward. Most of these people continue to suffer because cures are usually attempted with medication, whereas the cause is purely a mechanical one.

"Dr. Emanuel Josephson of New York City who wrote a commentary on my book said that pressures on the arm and shoulder during sleep can lead to bursitis. The cause is injury to the lubricating system of the shoulder. There is a delicate sac in the shoulder joint which is moistened by an oily fluid. Pressure on the shoulder muscle during sleep can in some cases cause a breakdown of its

Here are illustrations of the postures to avoid:

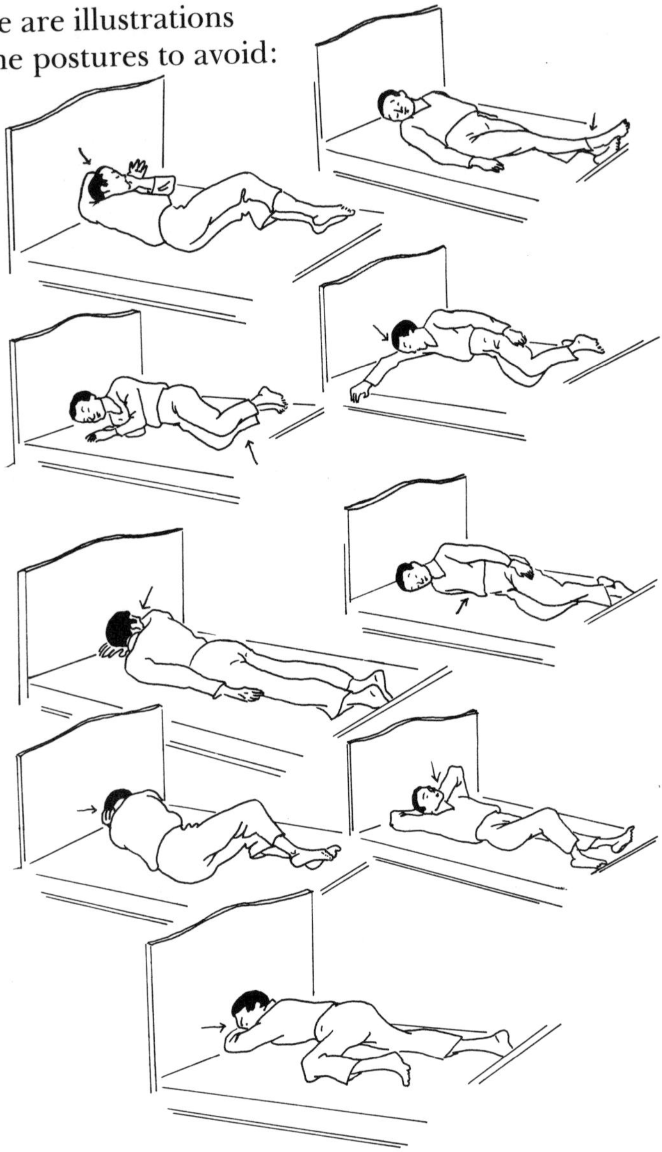

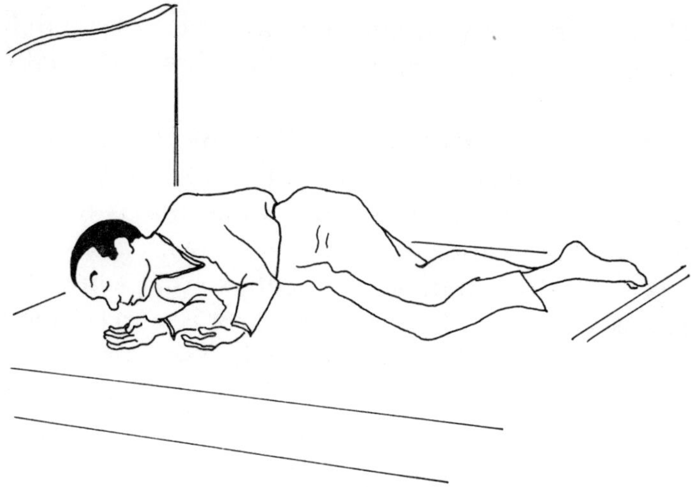

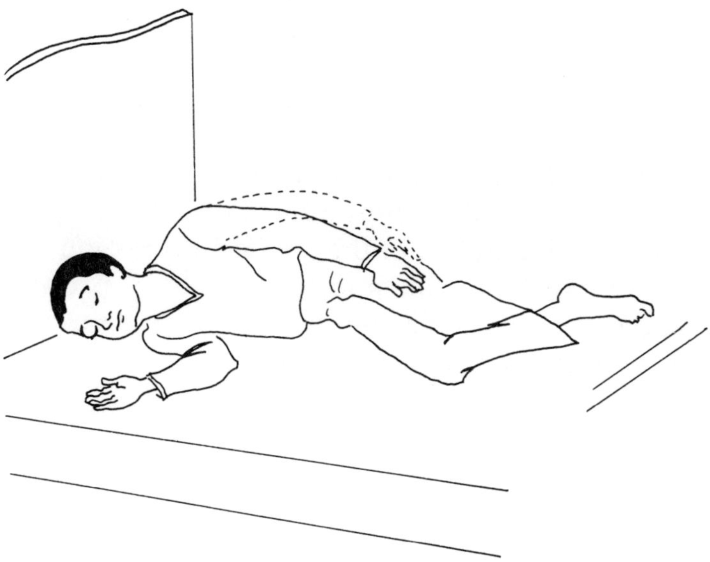

Here are illustrations of safe positions in sleep

lubricating system, giving rise to a case of subdeltoid bursitis and so many of these cases are usually operated on.

"Many a drunkard has fallen asleep in a hallway and because there are no pillows handy, used his arm for that purpose. But when one is drunk, the circulation and forces of the body are at even a lower ebb than in ordinary sleep, so that when the man is suddenly awakened, his arm is so paralyzed that he can hardly move it. Such cases sometimes have to be hospitalized, and in the big cities so many of them are brought into hospitals that this condition has been called Saturday Night Neuritis, from the fact that so many workers are paid at the end of the week, indulging in wild bouts of drinking and sleeping it off under tables, etc.

"Yet, though the doctors have handled so many of these drunkards, and knew that it came from sleeping on their arms, they did not think to associate it with other cases of arm neuritis. You can search high and low in the medical profession and nary a word will you find that the head pressing on the arm in sleep is the cause of these thousands of cases of pressure neuritis."

CHAPTER XIV

Sciatica

ALTHOUGH FEW PEOPLE realize it, sciatica—that infamous pain which can occur anywhere from the lower back to the feet—is actually one form of neuritis. By the term sciatica, we mean pain which originates in the sciatic nerve or branches of it.

In the February, 1960, issue of *The Practitioner,* R. A. Henson, M.D., makes the point that "The diagnosis of sciatica should be made with care. There is a tendency to use the term for all pains radiating from the lumbar region or buttock down the lower limb. This is a dangerous assumption. Pain may be felt down the thigh in disease of the pelvic bones and in affections of the hip or sacro-iliac joints. A safe rule to adopt is to regard pains radiating from the back or buttock down the back or outside of the thigh to below the midcalf as sciatic, at the same time remembering that sciatic pain may not radiate this far. Difficulty is sometimes encountered in patients with two disease processes operating together to produce pains in the lower limbs. A familiar example is that of the elderly patient with osteoarthritis of the hip and arterial insufficiency in the lower limbs. A sophisticated approach is required to distinguish the two components, joint and ischaemic pains. The unwary may mistake them for the one pain of an attack of sciatica."

What Henson is saying, in effect, is that all backaches and pain of the lower limbs are not sciatic in nature, and that the physician must be sure to make the distinction. Most of these ailments are very serious regarding their causation. Sciatica, while less dangerous, can be excruciatingly painful and should be promptly diagnosed.

Except in the rarest cases, the pain in sciatica is not due to an irritation to the sciatic nerve itself, experts believe. They say that the pain is referred to this area from nerve roots which could have been damaged due to such widely diverse reasons as a slipped disc, tuberculosis of the bone, vascular injuries which affected the spinal cord, meningitis and syphilis. The degree of pain varies with the patient, but in the worst cases the victim may be unable to stand or walk due to pain. Sneezing or coughing, or any sudden movements or jolting of the spine, can aggravate the irritation, and cause searing pain. Sitting or lying can be as uncomfortable as standing, so it is not surprising that serious sciatica victims are ready to do anything for relief, including submitting to surgery.

The surgical treatment is intended to correct a misplacement of a vertebra due to a loss of support by the disc which then causes the spinal column to list to one side. This results in the nerve's being pinched and the pain we sometimes call sciatica follows from that. One of two courses is usually followed in the surgery employed to alleviate this situation: the surgeon may place a support between the vertebrae to keep them the proper distance apart, or he might "fuse" the spinal column so that it cannot bend to either side at that point, and needs no support to keep it from leaning and closing the gap between the vertebrae.

For over one hundred years, the major controversy in treating sciatica has been whether or not long-term bed rest is desirable. Two researchers, Hilton and Thomas, are the classical exponents of this therapy—and they advocate it with such zeal that they overlook the serious side effects of it.

Danish researcher E. Schack Staffeldt wrote an interesting account of prolonged bed rest in sciatica as compared to an exercise program. The following excerpts are taken from that article, which appeared in *Ugesk. laeger,* February 25, 1960:

"One group consisted of 100 patients with the sciatica syndrome who were in the medical department of the Aarhus Hospital from September, 1949 to April, 1951. . . .

"The author has examined all patients on admittance, followed them regularly during their stay and finally made the dismissal examination.

"For comparison 100 patients were used who were admitted to the same place in the period from 1938 to 1942, and all were diagnosed as having sciatica. The treatment of these patients had been prolonged, strictly enforced bed rest, heat treatments and massage but no exercises. The information about these patients comes entirely from their charts; their symptoms, ways of treatment together with the results are judged only from this chart information.

"Taking into account that these groups are not completely and directly comparable, it was thought that the results of the two different systematic treatments of sciatica patients is of interest.

"When in the actively treated cases no difference was made between patients with disc prolapse and those with disc pains, this was done for reasons of comparison, because no systematic difference was made among the patients from 1938 to 1942, who suffered a positive disc prolapse and sciatica syndrome from other causes. We chose to judge the results of the exercise during the period of 1949 to 1951, because the patients who received active treatment after 1951 had supplemental treatment such as local anesthesia, epidermal injections, stretch exercises and the like.

"For the judgment of the treatment effect the following criteria were used:

"1. How long was the hospital stay in the two groups?

"2. How long did it take for the Lasegue to become negative?

"3. How long did it take to get the patients free of pain and to calm down?

"4. When could the patients move freely without pain?

"Both groups consisted of 100 patients each, and there were 47 males and 53 females in the first group, and 55 males and 45 females in the second. . . .

"A rough average establishes a hospital stay of approximately 50 days for the passively treated group and approximately 30 days for the actively treated one. But the difference is too great to carry through a direct comparison. . . .

"The hospital stay for the passive group is much longer than for the actively treated one. Even if one would exclude the four patients in the 1938 group, who remained in the hospital the longest and who probably at the present time would be moved to a special department with an operation in view, there is still a clear cut difference in the hospital stay days. The criteria for dismissal have not been changed from the first group in 1938 and the patients are not dismissed in poor shape. . . the patients from 1949 were free of pain earlier than those of 1938.

"It should be mentioned here that the patients in the latter group, judging from the charts, were not more affected than those in the 1949-1951 group."

Dr. Staffeldt explained that the exercises must be such that they do not impose a strain on the spine. They began following one week of bed rest. (Staffeldt says, "No special beds were used and the patients did not have a wooden bedboard in the bed, because no proof was found that this was beneficial.")

Relaxing exercises are important, especially those which relax the leg and gluteal muscles. Staffeldt has the patients sit in the L-shape position to practice hip flexibility exercises and head flexibility exercises. Respiratory exercises are also practiced. A major purpose of these various procedures used is to make sure there are no adhesions forming in an injured spinal column. Resistance exercises were also practiced in order to build up and strengthen the muscles of the back.

Among the other methods of sciatic treatment which have met with some success, heat therapy is one of the most important. Various sophisticated instruments have been developed by physical therapists to concentrate heat onto certain portions of the body. Diathermy devices as well as radio-therapy devices have been used effectively. However, heating pads, hot water bottles or hot baths which an individual can use himself are cheaper, and according to some physicians, equally effective.

Finally, Burns and Young point out that sciatica often improves all by itself, even without any treatment whatsoever. They write, ". . . in a year even the severest attack of sciatica is likely to subside either completely or, less often, into a chronic grumbling ache in the back or thigh. Recurrent attacks of lumbago or sciatica also tend to improve, becoming less frequent and less severe."

The best advice seems to be an adaption of the old maxim "haste makes waste." In this case, haste may make for needless pain and suffering—especially when that haste is in the direction of surgery. Conservative therapy is in the vast majority of cases sufficient, and surgery should be resorted to only when the condition is so severe as to allow for no other course.

The Practitioner (February, 1960) schedules treatment for a severe disc injury in this way: bed rest for 14 days, with a fracture board under the mattress. Local heat should be applied to relieve pain. Non-weight-bearing exercise on lower limbs (lifting legs and moving them from side to side) on 10th day. Once the patient is considered recovered and is released, he should do no heavy work, and he may have to wear a cast or corset for support.

There is very little literature to be found on the use of food supplements as a therapeutic agent in treating sciatica. *The Vitamins in Medicine,* a book by Bicknell and Prescott, mentions that some researchers have claimed relief of sciatica through the use of thiamin, but that "these claims have never (up to 1953) been confirmed. . . ."

While no definite therapeutic effect was proven

with thiamin, we believe that diets rich in the B vitamins to strengthen the nerves, protein to build firm tissues which will properly place the disc and reinforce it and bone meal to strengthen the bones of the spine, and each vertebra in particular, can contribute much to the prevention of sciatica.

Apparently vitamin C can also help ease lower back pain including sciatica. Dr. James Greenwood, Jr. of Baylor University College of Medicine reported in the *Medical Annals of the District of Columbia* that vitamin C in large doses has helped patients with back, neck, or leg pain due to spinal disc injuries. Some patients, he reports, have been able to avoid the necessity for surgery and others have been able to avoid recurrence of the syndrome when their vitamin C intake was increased.

The relationship between vitamin C and the building of bones, blood vessels, cartilage and collagen has long been established. It was this relationship which prompted Dr. Greenwood to try vitamin C for his own personal stab in the back which had been keeping him at home on the heating pad for a period of 10 years while his pain grew sharper and more severe with each attack.

But four months after he started taking 100 milligrams of vitamin C three times a day he was comfortable and able to exercise without difficulty. As soon as he cut the vitamin C out of his daily schedule, he was back on the heating pad. When he resumed taking it, he improved.

Dr. Greenwood applied the benefits of his own

experience to more than 500 patients crippled with back pain and reports gratifying relief even when the pain was caused by a slipped disc.

"At present," Dr. Greenwood says, "we recommend 500 milligrams a day in two doses (250 milligrams each) with an increase to 1,000 milligrams if there is any discomfort or if heavy exercise, such as hunting, sailing, boating, etc. is anticipated."

Dr. Greenwood says that the official estimate of the need for vitamin C (10 to 20 milligrams daily) is based on the amount needed to prevent absolute scurvy, a severe deficiency. Actually a smaller deficiency might account for the spinal problems which have put him and millions of others flat on their heating pads, he says.

With the exception of man, monkeys, guinea pigs, the Indian fruit fly and the red vented bulbul, all species synthesize their own vitamin C and maintain their supply at saturation point in their tissues. Could this be why your pet dogs and cats don't get pains in their backs?

Dr. Greenwood reports that he has found no indication in the medical literature that any harm can come from large doses of ascorbic acid except when a patient is also taking steroid drugs such as cortisone and ACTH. (Vitamin C helps the body to manufacture its own steroid hormones.)

To help strengthen tissues and prevent degeneration, he says, "probably all of us ought to take more vitamin C."

CHAPTER XV

Bursitis

PERHAPS THE HOUSEWIFE is a little ambitious with the scrub brush. Perhaps she sweeps a little too hard. Or stretches a little too far washing the windows.

The man may take one too many overambitious strokes with a golf club or pound too hard with a hammer. A game of baseball or volleyball at the Sunday School Picnic can lead to it. The result is bursitis, one of the most painful ailments known to man.

Unfortunately, it is also one of the most common of the rheumatic diseases. It starts usually during middle age, more frequently in women than in men. In some professions, bursitis is a recognized occupational hazard. Baseball players, orchestra leaders, violinists and others who work the arm very hard, or hold it for long periods of time at difficult positions, experience bursitis so frequently that attacks of the ailment in certain locations can actually be named after the professions with which they are associated. The best example of this is tennis elbow.

There are about 140 bursas in the body. Bursas are closed sacs lined by connective tissue and containing a small amount of synovial fluid. The little sacs are usually located over bony prominences, especially those over which muscle or tendon moves. The reason for the bursas is to make it easy for the muscles or the tendons to glide over the bony structures and thereby reduce friction.

Sometimes, for one reason or another, some individuals will develop a bony protrusion in an area where most people do not have them. If there is friction when tendons or muscles move over that area, the body will automatically develop another bursa. Thus, although scientists have named, as we have said, about 140 bursas in the human being, most of us will have several others in areas rather unique to ourselves.

Any number of factors can irritate a bursa—so many, in fact, that it is a wonder the ailment is not even more widespread than it is. Any trauma—injury or irritation, from a physical source—can disturb a bursa. In fact, that is apparently the most frequent cause of bursitis. But sometimes a cut can also cause the disease by allowing staphylococcus, streptococcus, pneumococcus, or gonococcus organisms to enter the bursa and cause an infection. Rheumatic fever and allergies have produced bursitis, and so have tuberculosis, syphilis, salmonella and lead poisoning.

Although it is quite rare, even some forms of cancer can irritate the bursas and trigger off a case of bursitis.

What happens after the bursa is irritated through any one of those sources? The June, 1955, issue of *Today's Health* describes the process well:

"The first trace of irritation makes every tiny blood vessel in the bursa's wall fill itself to capacity with extra blood for fighting off the trouble. Thus engorged, these blood vessels transform the slick, bearing-like inner surface to harsh, sandpaper roughness. At every motion of the muscles or tendons it is lubricating, the bursa grates painfully. The trouble-fighting legions of the bloodstream pour forth on a wave of fluid, and the balloonlike bursa swells until its fragile walls are stretched beyond endurance. Its pleas for respite flood the switchboard of the pain nerves in the area. Not only does the bursa hurt; the whole arm or leg or shoulder hurts as nearby pain nerves echo the call."

Unless one is absolutely sure of what caused a bursitis attack, it is imperative that he seek a medical diagnosis to establish that information. Bursitis, painful as it is, can be a blessing if it leads to an early diagnosis of a serious disease causing it.

In the great majority of cases, bursitis results

from overuse of a limb, muscle or tendon. The result is that the bursa is irritated by constant friction. In these cases, treatment of the bursa alone is sufficient.

At one time, the medical community resorted to extremes in their attempts to treat bursitis. Surgery, as well as unnecessarily powerful drugs were used almost routinely. Even today, some doctors will use a strong narcotic for killing the pain and resort without hesitation to cortisone or—even less justifiable—x-ray. But, according to the June, 1955, *Today's Health,* ". . . Many doctors are switching to simple measures with good results."

One such measure mentioned in that publication is the use of heat: "By studying the actual temperature changes in and around inflamed tissue during treatment, a group of researchers has proved that it is more beneficial to heat the surface but cool the actual diseased area. Apparently, the old-fashioned idea of drawing congestion to the surface is not too far off in bursitis. At least, there's a good chance that much of the good done by heat treatment in joint inflammations and similar conditions comes from the dilation of surface channels, drawing off the fluid from the congested blood vessels in the area of the disease. This fits in with oft-proved fact that paraffin baths, hot soaks, and contrast baths (four minutes hot soak, one in cold, four more in heat, and so on ending with heat) gives more relief in many cases than any of the deep-heating machines."

Also praising the use of heat is the October 10, 1963, *New England Journal of Medicine.* According to the journal, "Local heat applied intermittently, half-an-hour out of every four, increases circulation locally and helps produce relaxation in the muscles in the affected area. The relief is temporary but may be quite effective, both in alleviating pain and in enabling exercises to be carried out more frequently during convalescence."

A number of mechanical devices are available to provide heat to certain areas of the body. Ordinary infrared or heat lamps are effective enough to cure mild cases. Many doctors have instruments which generate heat by passing radio waves through certain areas of the body. These devices, called diathermy machines, not only heat the skin surface, but generate heat through the entire tissue including the irritating bursa. Newer machines use ultra short sound waves which apparently also produce heat. Some authorities say these are at least as effective as the radio wave devices.

Immediately after a bursitis attack, especially a very severe one, the *Journal* points out that affected limbs should be immobilized with a splint and sling. The idea is to not irritate the bursa at all for a while so that natural body healing processes can go to work effectively (in very, very serious cases, the *Journal* also recommends a new drug, phenylbutazone, which has had considerable success in treating bursitis. The *Journal* points out, however, that the drug is not to be given to patients with a history of ulcers—and as a matter of policy, drugs should never be taken, except as a last resort when the pain is unbearable.)

This therapy is so successful that, the *Journal* says, a dramatic response occurs in most cases within 48 to 72 hours—and occasionally even within 24 hours. There is a rapid loss of pain and increase in available motion.

As soon as motion returns and pain lessens, exercise is absolutely essential. That point is made in the October 15, 1951, *Modern Medicine.* "All forms of treatment are supplemented by exercise, consisting of wall climbing, external rotation, stretching the arms behind the head, hourly pendulum and circumduction motions, and internal stretching behind the back," says *Modern Medicine.* The publication warns that if six or eight weeks pass before exercises are undertaken, the arm may be stiffly immobilized. This will require hospital care or daily physical therapy. The situation can be avoided—and certainly ought to be—by beginning even the simplest of exercises as soon as possible after an attack. Such simple procedures as merely swinging the arm gently back and forth at the side, or using the opposite arm to assist in bringing the affected one overhead or behind the back are adequate at first. However, as the *New England Journal* points out, "Short periods of frequent exercise are the rule." When not exercising, and especially at night, the limb should be carefully protected against any unconscious movement or pressure.

Bursitis and Exercise

J. I. Rodale found that an exercise bicycle provided good exercise therapy for bursitis. The motion of this machine—the Exercycle—forced his arms into a rhythmic exercise pattern as he gripped the handle bars and loosened tense muscles.

In the December, 1962 issue of *Prevention,* Mr. Rodale described another case in which exercise offered a cure for bursitis: "A taxi driver in New York City last week told me of a friend of his who was afflicted with bursitis in his shoulder for many years. The doctors could do nothing for him. He was cured by taking up bowling. We know that when a person is inactive, his glands do not function well, to make all the hormones needed in the various body processes. Any exercise, especially bowling, makes the body work on all its cylinders. I would say also that bowling, by oxygenating the body, can do a lot of good, besides the incidental curing of a case of bursitis.

"I asked the cabby whether bowling was not a one-sided thing, favoring only one side of the body and he replied that if I watched bowlers I would see that both sides are exercised. One of these days I will go to a bowling alley."

Needless to say if the bursitis has been caused by any overuse or stress, that sort of activity should be avoided after one has recuperated from a bursitis attack. Also important is that one should gradually warm up to any physical activity using the limb. It is no more sensible to engage in a strenuous game of tennis without first warming up the limbs and getting the blood to circulate through them freely than it would be to start your automobile engine on a wintery morning and immediately participate in a drag race.

One of several books containing a good deal of information on bursitis is *Arthritis—What to do About It* by Robert D. Potter, Executive Secretary of the Medical Society of New York. In it he mentions all of the standard methods the medical profession has developed for treating bursitis. But what stands out in Potter's book is not so much what he does say as what he doesn't say. There is, for example, nothing at all in his book on the effect diet may have on this disease. However, the question is brought up rather obliquely in an article by N. W. Paul, abstracted in the *Journal of the American Medical Association* for November 30, 1957. In a report on 314 patients with so-called "tennis elbow" (radiohymeral bursitis), evidence was found that the primary cause was neither injury nor occupation but a metabolic disturbance. Or, in other words, the body either wasn't using its food efficiently, or it wasn't getting the proper food in the first place. This inability of the body to use its food properly was reduced to two possible causes by the author: either nervous or hormonal disturbance. To correct this he orders all emotional tension and stimulants to the nervous system be reduced. Physical therapy is not suggested —and an antipurine diet is recommended. This diet is based upon Dr. Paul's theory that too much uric acid is present in the bloodstream, as in gout, and that foods containing this acid should be discontinued. These foods are chiefly meats, especially organ meats.

We are forced to disagree with Dr. Paul in this instance. While we believe that the excess of uric acid is caused, as Dr. Paul says, by faulty metabolism, if the body's mechanics are inefficient, they are likely to be so if even the smaller amount of uric acid is eaten. Straighten out the metabolism, we say, but give the body the natural foods it needs. And the very meats that Dr. Paul prohibits are rich in the vitamins which help to regulate the metabolism.

In support of this view we cite an article appearing in *Industrial Medicine and Surgery,* June, 1957, by Dr. I. S. Klemes, Medical Director of the Ideal Mutual Insurance Company and J. C. Penny Company in New York City. Since 1953 Dr. Klemes has been treating subdeltoid bursitis (shoulder bursitis) with vitamin B_{12} and has had great success.

Dr. Klemes gives several case histories to illustrate the effectiveness of vitamin B_{12} in dealing with bursitis. A typical one will serve our purpose here: An executive was encountered as he rested, baking under an infrared lamp in the hot summer of 1955. He was there at his own request. He had all the clinical signs of acute subdeltoid bursitis—pain and marked restriction in movement of the shoulder, plus tenderness over the bursa. The patient refused to have an x-ray and was not favorable to a series of vitamin B_{12} injections. When he returned three days later, he was in marked pain. He was in such pain that he agreed to the procedure suggested to him before. X-rays showed an appreciable amount of callus in the subdeltoid bursa. He experienced relief within a few hours after the first injection of vitamin B_{12}. The relief continued steadily and in five days the man was symptom free. He was able to move his arm above shoulder level. X-rays taken six weeks later showed definite absorption of callus, and there has been no return of symptoms since; functional restoration has remained complete.

This course of treatment has been effective for Dr. Klemes in all types of bursitis cases. In the five years it has been used, only three of Dr. Klemes' cases have not responded. Certainly it is worth trying in place of cortisone, nerve blocks and surgery! The relief is rapid, calcium deposits, if any, are absorbed; there are no side effects and overdosage is almost impossible. There is no definite site for the injections and they are given as follows: Daily doses of 1 cc. or 1,000 mcg. of vitamin B_{12} for seven to 10 days, then three times per week for two or three weeks. Then one or two a week for two or three weeks, depending upon clinical indications. Also important is the fact that the treatment is relatively inexpensive compared with x-ray and hormone treatments.

Of course, many doctors will pooh-pooh Dr. Klemes' work, and simply refuse to try it, preferring to rely on the dangerous, and often ineffective methods they're used to. We think that ignoring this method of treatment, even on the sheerest possibility that it may work is most unwise.

Klemes' theories on vitamin B_{12} are in agreement with an article from the *Journal of the American Medical Association* (June, 1956) in which the authors noted these facts about folic acid and vitamin B_{12}. "Vitamin B_{12} and folic acid both seem to be essential in the synthesis of nucleoproteins. . . . It seems certain that vitamin B_{12} is of importance in the metabolism of nervous tissue, although the mechanism of its action is not known . . . Vitamin B_{12} has proved effective in relieving the pain of trigeminal neuralgia in a significant proportion of patients." So there you have an unbiased basis for Dr. Klemes' work. Note, too, that the article from the *Journal* says vitamin B_{12} is important in regulating metabolism. Now if you omit meats and organ meats from your diet, chances are you will not be getting any vitamin B_{12} at all, as it is most abundant in these foods. So an anti-purine diet would be almost certainly a diet completely lacking in vitamin B_{12}.

Maybe readers not yet plagued by bursitis, can save themselves from the problem by eating regularly of foods rich in the elements which make bursitis disappear, foods rich in B vitamins. These are brewer's yeast, wheat germ, liver (desiccated liver or whole) and other organ meats. Preventing a shortage of B vitamins will probably keep you bursitis-free, and free from a number of other physical problems too.

Vitamin C is another nutritional element that should not be ignored in cases of bursitis. We know this vitamin to be effective in similar diseases such as arthritis, so why not give it a try in licking bursitis? We printed a letter a few years ago from one of our Canadian readers, Mrs. W. C. Godfrey of Duchess, Alberta, Canada. She wrote this: "You may be interested in the fact that after my husband took rose hips powder (loaded with vitamin C) for three or four months, his bursitis left him and has not returned." Remember, please, that rose hips or any other natural form of vitamin C is not exactly the same as synthetic vitamin C which you buy at the drug store. The natural food source contains the bioflavonoids and no one knows how big a part these play in the results you get from using a natural food supplement as your source of vitamin C.

Don't discount the role of nutrition in illness. Perhaps a review of dietary habits and a reinforcement of your body's nutritional supply will spare you the pain, money and time wasted in treating a rheumatic type of illness by some other method that can only hope to relieve, not cure, you.

CHAPTER XVI

Back Pain

THE National Safety Council estimates disabling back ailments afflicting millions of Americans cost the economy well over $1 billion annually in lost goods and services. Workmen's compensation payments amount to nearly $225 million for some 234,540 back injury cases, according to the council. And the organization feels the actual impact on the economy is at least four times the direct cost.

A United States Department of Health, Education and Welfare survey discloses most back and spine injuries happen on the job—35.5 per cent. Injuries at home, mostly from falls and lifting, run second at 23.2 per cent. Moving vehicle mishaps cause 22.6 per cent of injuries reported.

For the working man, such a disability often is as painful in the lower region of the billfold as in the spine. For example, the average Pennsylvanian in 1965 spent 73.31 days off the job at a cost of $485.83. The average Florida resident suffered through 108.53 days away from work at a loss of $835.83. American Chiropractic Association statistics reveal average per capita disability costs in 1965 ranged from $130.08 in South Carolina to a staggering $1,840.40 in New York.

If you are one of the millions of Americans who after physical exertion reacts with lower back pains—the all-inclusive heading of the diseases is lumbago—you are certainly not alone. Medical authorities estimate that one out of every two Americans eventually has that problem.

The general term used to summarize any backache is lumbago. *Dorland's Medical Dictionary* defines lumbago as "pain in the lumbar (low back) region; backache." Thus, any backache, but particularly that in the lower region, may correctly be termed lumbago. By that very broad definition, even sciatica, which we have dealt with previously in a separate chapter, can be fitted into this category if the pain it produces occurs in the back. In such cases, lumbago may be an indication of a very serious ailment. But pressure on the sciatic nerve is only one of many possible causes of lumbago. Others, not all of them associated with the rheumatic diseases, include: an injury, a torn muscle or a misplaced vertebra.

If you are suffering from back pain, Dr. Von Walter Mohing gives this advice in the March 19,

1965, German medical journal, *Munchener Medizinische Wochenschrift:* First, eliminate the possibility of sciatica. Then, check for degenerative disease, tumors and other serious conditions. Although these things are rare, they are also serious. To ignore the possibility of their existence is not only foolish but potentially deadly.

Once these serious diseases are eliminated, Mohing gives the following advice regarding therapy:

"The therapy is mainly conservative; operative measures . . . are exceptions and are justified only after indication has carefully been established and after failure of thorough conservative treatment. Conservative treatment begins with intensive heat application, infiltration of the dorsal muscles to disrupt the arch of pain . . . it is followed later by massages and active physical exercise.—A level position on a hard base contributes to decrease the irritation. Supporting corsets may effectively complete the treatment of certain patients." Mohing also recommends certain drugs designed to relieve pain.

Any operation dealing with the spine is obviously a very serious procedure. All the nerves of the body's sympathetic nervous system run through the spinal cord, and when that cord is severed, the body is permanently paralyzed. Surgery is rarely necessary in lumbago.

Intensive heat application is frequently very effective in reducing pain and irritation. Massages, which also build up the body's heat in the particular area, work to reduce pain in the same way. In addition, massages relax tense muscles—and muscles that are very tense cause almost as much pain as the vertebrae themselves.

The exercise Dr. Mohing mentions is of particular importance. Combined with postural habits, exercise is probably the most important word in the vocabulary of any lumbago sufferer. As Dr. Hans Kraus, consultant to the late President John F. Kennedy, put it at an Industrial Medical Association Convention in New York City:

—More than 80 per cent of pain in the lower back is muscular in origin.

—Muscular imbalance producing pain is usually general, or postural, rather than due to local defects of the bones or joints.

—Muscular imbalances producing lower back pain are principally due to lack of exercise. Every general medical examination should include testing of the mobility and strength of muscles supporting the spine.

Dr. Kraus, associate professor of physical medicine at New York University's School of Medicine, said that the first episode of relatively mild low back pain is an excellent opportunity for the doctor to persuade his patient to take more active exercise.

George R. Bruce, weight training director of the Mid Valley YMCA in Van Nuys, California, also reminds back sufferers that every movement of the body is dependent upon its muscles. "It is the function of the muscles to hold the body and its contents in proper shape and in proper place,"

Bruce emphasized. "The stronger the muscles, the more easily they can carry on their designated functions."

In other words, lower back pain boils down to lack of exercise, weak muscles, lack of proper body shape, deterioration or lordosis, resultant strain on the spine, disc lesions or pressure on the nerve-crammed spinal cord. Any of those factors, alone or in combination, can cause the excruciating experience known as lower back pain. Most of them, according to Dr. Miland E. Knapp of the University of Minnesota's Medical School in Minneapolis, are curable. Treatments prescribed by Dr. Knapp include (in the acute stage) bed rest, support by taping or traction, hot packs, whirlpool baths, the Hubbard tank, aspirin, codeine, selected sedatives and manipulation.

"Probably the most important procedure for relieving low back pain during the acute stage is bed rest on a firm mattress over a bed board that covers the entire surface of the spring," Dr. Knapp writes. "A firm felt mattress is preferable, but a sponge rubber mattress with a compression ratio of 34 pounds per square inch is satisfactory and may be a little more comfortable."

Pelvic belts, corsets and heat have proven of value in relieving pain. Moist heat appears to be most useful when muscle spasm accompanies the pain. Traction is important, too, because muscle contractures often cause prolonged disability.

During subacute and chronic stages, exercises may be used to strengthen weak muscles. Writes

Dr. Knapp: "We usually start with postural exercises, stressing back-flattening if lordosis is present and adapting the program to fit the presenting symptoms. If weakness is severe, the best method of producing hypertrophy is progressive resistance exercises."

Probably more than 90 per cent of workers return to their jobs following back injury, and only a small percentage require surgical treatment. "Work Hardening Units," similar to one developed at the Minneapolis Curative Workshop, are often helpful in preparing patients and tender backs for the rigors of an eight-hour factory or office routine again.

Under the direction of the occupational therapist, a work program is set up which simulates as closely as possible the expected work situation. That may involve shoveling sand, lifting bricks and cement blocks, pushing a wheelbarrow, sawing or running a lathe. The patient visits the unit daily, working within his physical capacities until he can work through a six-hour day. He is then discharged, presumably sufficiently rehabilitated to assume his normal responsibilities.

Among key "Rules to Live By—From Now On," published by McNeil Laboratories of Fort Washington, Pennsylvania, are:

1. Never bend from the waist only; bend the hips and knees.

2. Never lift a heavy object higher than your waist.

3. Always face the object you wish to lift.

4. Avoid carrying unbalanced loads; hold heavy objects close to your body.

5. Never carry anything heavier than you can manage with ease.

6. Never move or lift heavy furniture. Wait for someone who knows the principles of leverage.

7. Avoid sudden movements, sudden "overloading" of muscles. Learn to move deliberately, swinging the legs from the hips.

8. Learn to keep the head in line with the spine, when standing, sitting, lying in bed.

9. Put soft chairs and deep couches on your "don't sit" list. During prolonged sitting, cross legs to rest your back.

10. Your doctor is the only one who can determine when low back pain is due to faulty posture. He is the best judge of when you may do physical exercises for physical fitness. When you do, omit any exercise which arches or overstrains the lower back: backward or forward bends, or touching the toes with the knees straight.

Most of these rules are actually rules of good posture—and good posture is extremely important in recovering from lumbago. But it is equally important in preventing lumbago in the first place. Joints, muscles and bones are the parts of the body which suffer most from poor posture.

What is the importance of posture in the prevention of lumbago? Good posture is essential for good health and it is especially important in any disorder in which bones, joints and muscles are involved, for these are the parts of the body which suffer most from bad posture.

Dr. B. T. Bell of Abington Memorial Hospital, writing on "The Diagnosis and Treatment of Low Back Pain," in the *Medical Clinics of North America* for November, 1940, says that the assumption of upright posture by man, with the resulting angulation, the systems of balance and leverage necessary to hold this upright posture, is one of the main reasons why the lower back is so susceptible to strain. The muscles of the lower back also seem to be insufficient to perform their work in the anatomy of mankind.

Says Dr. Bell, "Sedentary occupations or manual occupations in which the worker remains seated all day together with poor habits of posture result in a back which is barely compensating. A strain of lifting, or a fall, an excessive increase in weight or even increased weight-bearing will increase the load so that the symptoms of strain or more serious injury result. An illness resulting in further loss of muscle power may be the cause of insufficiency in the muscles and strain. In the back subjected to continued mild strain, chronic irritation increases the changes which appear as osteoarthritis in later life. . . . Often the patient with postural defects of flat feet, lumbar lordosis (swayback), sagging abdomen and obesity is symptom-free until some trauma (injury) is literally the last straw on the camel's back."

Doctors agree on the importance of good posture. They also agree that the individual determination to achieve good posture can work wonders, even though there are some postural handicaps that cannot be overcome without the aid of professional therapy. Perfect posture is so simple that there can be no disagreement as to what it means. It means keeping one's body in balance so that there is as little strain as possible on muscles, bones and nerves, when one stands, sits, walks or works.

The base of support for one's body is the pelvic structure—that is, the bony basin to which one's legs are attached, and which contains the abdominal organs.

The next time you are standing on a street corner waiting for someone, look at the people who pass. You will notice that bad posture can completely ruin an otherwise attractive appearance; you will see that tasteful and expensive clothes look like rags when the framework beneath them is sagging and out of balance. If you wait on your corner long enough, perhaps someone may come along who has a good posture. He will look relaxed, rested, healthy. There will be a spring to his step and a buoyancy in his appearance that will make you feel good just to look at him.

When you get home, take a look at yourself in a full-length mirror. Just stand naturally, as you usually stand. How do you look? Be honest with yourself. Then decide to do something to improve your posture. It won't be easy. If your body has accustomed itself to frightfully bad posture, you will have to do a lot of coaxing to regain good posture for by this time bones, muscles and nerves have gotten set in this bad pattern.

The first and, yes, we might say, the only exercise necessary to begin correcting the commonest off-balance posture, is to pull in on the muscles of your abdomen. It's just as simple as that. The curve in the back straightens out, which in turn corrects the flat chest and rounded shoulders. As these fall into line, the legs and feet assume their rightful positions and good posture becomes a reality.

However, if your posture is really sagging, you'll find that it's not easy to pull in your stomach muscles. They're flabby and soft from disuse. Try again the second day and the third. It may take weeks before you notice the slightest improvement in the trimness of your figure. You don't have to set aside any time for exercise if you want to have good posture. Just fit it into your daily regime. You can practice good posture while you are waiting for a trolley, standing in an elevator, talking on the telephone.

Housework involves a large percentage of us, so let's discuss posture in terms of housework. While you're getting breakfast in the morning, waiting for the eggs to boil, check on your posture. Pull in your tummy and tuck your lower back under where it belongs. Now see how you can improve posture and ward off fatigue while you're working. When you bend to pick something up, to reach something or to do some particular kind of work, bend at your knees or hips—don't bend your back. No matter how you manage to do it, see that your sink, stove, laundry tubs and other working spaces are at exactly the right height for you—not so high that you must stretch to reach them, not so low that you must bend or stoop. Sitting is better than standing at any job where it can possibly be managed. Until you've tried sitting while you iron, you won't realize how much energy you can save this way. Sit down in the kitchen while you're preparing vegetables, sit down to wash the dishes. Make sure your chair is comfortable and that you are sitting with your back straight, your stomach muscles pulled in. Be certain you have support for your feet, check from time to time to make sure your shoulders are back, but relaxed, so that you are not "humped" tensely over your work.

You can exercise for good posture while you are making a bed, sweeping a floor, setting a table, running a sewing machine. If you remember only one basic commandment—keep your stomach muscles pulled in—the rest of your body will align itself properly. Have you ever estimated how much time you spend each week walking to and from stores carrying packages? Have you ever stopped to think how important to your posture the way in which you carry those packages is? At your dressing table mirror you can check on your shoulders. When you are standing as you normally do, one is probably higher than the other, for no other reason but that, since you were in school, you have become accustomed to carrying books, purse, umbrella, packages always in the same arm. In most people this practice results in carrying the shoulder of that arm as much as several inches higher than the other shoulder—bad posture. This throws the whole upper part of your body out of line and somewhere your bones and muscles must compensate, resulting in a lot of wear and tear, which you might easily avoid by simply remembering to carry equal weights in both arms or by shifting the weight from side to side.

Actually the only hard thing about regaining good posture is reminding yourself of it. Once the muscles have been strengthened, you'll have good posture without giving it another thought. But meanwhile, make a habit of studying your reflection in shop windows when you're walking on the street. One glance will remind you to pull those stomach muscles in. At home or at work decide on some one object—a calendar, a window, a piece of furniture that will be your constant reminder every time you look at it to correct your posture. You may be saving yourself years of agonizing pain with lumbago later on in life.

In Conclusion: Great Days Ahead

We are standing on the threshold of the greatest scientific era man has ever known. Human beings are reaching the bottom of the deepest seas, walking on the moon, building chains of skyscrapers across continents and learning nature's most intimate secrets.

The knowledge explosion today is fantastic beyond anything mankind has ever comprehended. In medicine the result is man's ability to prevent scores of diseases which once were fatal to multitudes. Among them are scarlet fever, the plague and polio. We have also learned how to prevent certain forms of cancer and heart disease, and while hundreds of thousands still die of these diseases each year, at least we have the knowledge, if it will be applied, to save a considerable number of those lives.

It may, in fact, be said that science in the second half of this decade has actually begun to "come of age." In previous years, the scientific community could be compared to a brilliant adolescence—many bright, creative ideas, but headstrong, impetuous, naive and self-centered to the point of blindness to reality. Pesticides were the miracle answer to crop-destroying insects. (No thought could be given to the possibility that pesticides themselves could cause harm.) Industrialization and the automobile staining the horizon with pollutants were impeccable symbols of progress and anyone who offered the slightest criticism was a right-wing radical. Drugs were meant to save lives, and anyone who found fault with them had to be a food faddist or a nut.

Today, science and scientists are on the threshold of maturity. It is common knowledge that pesticides do carry with them some very serious potential hazards—not only to wildlife, but to man himself. Everyone including the federal government is much concerned over disease-causing air pollution. The American Medical Association runs a regular feature on the adverse effects of drugs. Today, science has come to realize that technology and chemistry and the products produced therefrom, while useful, are by no means the be-all and end-all. Biological reality dare not be ignored.

These facts have given rise to a new concept of medicine—biological medicine. One of the major contentions of biological medicine is that, given ideal circumstances, the body can maintain optimum health or heal itself when illness develops. Chemistry and technology must not be forced upon biological processes.

According to this new concept, virtually every ailment—including arthritis and the rheumatic diseases—can indeed be cured. The miracle is not performed by a doctor or by a drug or even by supernatural intervention. The physician practicing biological medicine simply tries to determine what factor or factors in an ideal biological environment is not present in the case of his patient. He then attempts to establish the ideal environment which will give the body an opportunity to heal. Sometimes that may mean increasing certain nutrients, the fuel which the body uses to carry on its normal functions. It may mean something to increase the body's temperature, especially in the afflicted area, where temperature increase is one of the means whereby the body helps to fight disease.

This book has been devoted to presenting the latest information available on how, primarily through natural biological methods, doctors around the world have had success treating the arthritic and rheumatic diseases. It is still true that orthodox medicine recognizes no cure for these ailments. Yet, the doctors who have used methods presented in this book as compared to the costly and often dangerous drugs now being promoted by pharmaceutical manufacturers, attest that they have had far more success than the orthodox practitioners can claim. They deserve an open-minded hearing rather than defeatist scoffing.

Must you really go on suffering everlasting pain? Let the ideas in this book guide you to possible relief and perhaps in some cases cure. You have every reason to be hopeful. For, as the many cases cited in this book indicate, you are not alone in your suffering, but improvement and cure have come for many, and might for you too.

INDEX

-A-

-B-

-C-

-D-

-E-

-F-

-G-

INDEX

-H-

-I-

-J-

-K-

-L-

-M-

-N-

-O-

-P-

-R-

-S-

INDEX

-T-

-U-

-V-

-W-